W9-CLY-853

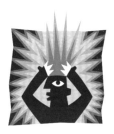

Headaches
A Cleveland Clinic Handbook

Robert S. Kunkel, M.D., F.A.C.P.

Cleveland Clinic Press

Cleveland, Ohio

Headaches: A Cleveland Clinic Handbook

Contact:

Cleveland Clinic Press

9500 Euclid Avenue NA32, Cleveland, Ohio 44195

216-445-5547 / delongk@ccf.org

www.clevelandclinicpress.org

This book is not intended to replace personal medical care and supervision; there is no substitute for the experience and information that your doctor can provide. Rather, this book seeks to provide useful information on the nature and diagnosis of headaches.

Proper medical care should always be tailored to the individual patient. If you read something in this book that seems to conflict with your doctor's instructions, contact your doctor. Since individual cases differ, there may be good reasons for individual treatment to differ from the information presented in this book.

If you have any questions about any suggestion made in this book, consult your doctor.

The patient names and cases used in this book do not represent actual people but are composite cases drawn from several sources.

Library of Congress Cataloging-in-Publication Data

Kunkel, Robert S.

Headaches: A Cleveland Clinic Handbook / Robert S. Kunkel.

p. cm.

Includes index.

ISBN 978-1-59624-019-3 (alk. paper)

1. Headache--Popular works.   I. Title.

RB128.K86 2007   616.8'491--dc22

2007020070

Cover design: J. Michael Myers • Book design: Meredith Pangrace
Drawings: Ken Kula (pp. 10-12), Joe Kanasz (p. 26), Cleveland Clinic Center for Medical Art and Photography

Cover illustration: "My Grain of Hope," by Marion Pruitt. This image and those depicted on pages 45-48 are used with permission of the National Headache Foundation.
For more information on headache causes and treatments, visit www.headaches.org.

Introduction

Headache is one of the common maladies suffered by human beings. Almost everyone has had a headache at some time in his or her life. There are millions who suffer with recurring, severe, disabling headaches. In my forty-plus years of caring for headache patients, I have seen much advancement in the knowledge and understanding of why people have pain in the head. While the underlying mechanisms of head pain are still not completely understood, it is now apparent that migraine, cluster, and many "tension-type" headaches are due to periodic or chronic dysfunction of neurons (brain cells) in the brain. Repetitive impulses from the brain go over nerves that branch out to the blood vessels, muscles, scalp, and other structures of the head. These nerves become overactive and hypersensitive, causing pain in their area of distribution.

The vast majority of headaches are of the "primary" type (migraine, cluster, and tension-type) and are not due to serious diseases such as brain tumors, infections, and aneurysms. Sinus disease is a rare cause of recurring headaches, yet many people feel that their headaches are due to "sinus" because the pain is in the front of their heads. The best way to make the correct diagnosis is with a good history of the headache characteristics, triggers, and any associated symptoms. Testing with CAT scans or MRI scans is not necessary to diagnose most headaches, but in order to exclude any possible underlying brain disease, which might be a factor in the pain, these studies are important.

The medical profession is becoming increasingly interested in headache and other chronic pain conditions. Today there are many more pain clinics and headache clinics than existed just a few years ago. More people are being trained in the specialties of pain management and headache medicine. A number of effective medications are now available to ease the pain and suffering of recurring headaches, and so are a variety of nonpharmacological treatments. Persons with headaches should not have to continue to suffer with chronic pain!

Organizations such as the National Headache Foundation and numerous websites offer valuable information and resources for the headache sufferer. (See Resources, page 111.) Despite the increase in available information and help, surveys have shown that about 50 percent of those in the United States who are living with migraine headaches have never consulted a professional for their headache problem. Many continue to suffer and lose days of productivity without the benefit of effective treatment.

This book is a handy resource for people dealing with chronic headaches. In it, I describe the most common types of headaches, their characteristics, some of the triggers that may be factors, and many of the effective treatments available.

Robert S. Kunkel, M.D.
Fellow of the American College of Physicians

Contents

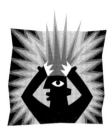

Chapter 1
Defining Headache

When Delores calls in sick with one of her frequent headaches, her colleagues roll their eyes and trade unsympathetic remarks around the fax machine. "It's just a headache," they say with a shrug. "She should get a grip on herself and come to work."

Delores is one of more than 45 million Americans who suffer from chronic recurring headaches. Their symptoms are often dismissed as psychosomatic or "all in their heads," but the fact is that chronic headaches are legitimate health complaints that wreak havoc in sufferers' lives.

Tension-type headaches are the most common headaches among both children and adults. However, migraine and cluster headaches are usually much more debilitating. Twenty-eight million Americans suffer from migraine. Cluster headaches, which can be 100 times more intense than migraines, affect about 1 million people – and those who love them – in the United States.

The toll of headaches

Migraine sufferers alone lose more than 150 million workdays each year. Industry loses an estimated $50 billion per year to absenteeism, lost productivity, and medical expenses caused by headaches.

Headaches cause more than a productivity problem in the workplace. They can take a terrible toll on the entire family. Consider the fact that one in four U.S. households includes a migraine sufferer. Yet more than half of those living with migraines have never been diagnosed.

Too many people with headaches don't seek help. They may know that one of their parents suffered from headaches and just accept their condition without question, treating it as their parents did years ago – by taking an over-the-counter medication and lying down. But with a variety of effective medications now available to treat and prevent headaches, the chance of success with one of these preventive medications is good.

Headaches may be a misunderstood and underappreciated problem, but they are legitimate illnesses that can be treated.

Making an electronic connection

Numerous support groups for headache sufferers exist around the country. Pen Pals, a successful program of the National Headache Foundation, puts folks with similar headaches together online to chat.

In this day of electronic communications, Internet blogs, or free personal websites, one can find new outlets where headache sufferers can post their pain and commiserate with fellow sufferers, talk about new findings (medical and otherwise), and alert each other to fraudulent headache-remedy claims.

Most of all, these online diaries help sufferers to realize that they are not alone. And they're good places for friends and family members to get a better understanding of a loved one's pain.

One blogger writes that the reason so many people are creating a public record is because they're trying to explain to themselves and to the world how debilitating and life-altering chronic headaches can be:

"Most people, when they think of headaches, think of a mildly annoying pain that makes you a little grumpy, lasts for an hour or two, and can be relieved with an Excedrin. For those of us with frequent cluster headaches or migraines, it can really feel like no one understands or, worse yet,

assumes you're faking, exaggerating, or simply not 'brave' or 'tough.'"

Frustrations of another cluster sufferer, once a very independent man, show through in this recent Internet blog entry:

"The worst part of clusters is being trapped inside one's body. I have come to the realization that without the aid of others, I would be in big trouble, and I hate it. I need to be driven everywhere. A job is out of the question. Who would be willing to hire someone who will be in pain 360 out of 365 days a year, not be able to guarantee that they will be able to show up for work when scheduled, or have to leave when the pain becomes intolerable?"

Other sufferers describe their desperation:

"There are times when this disease overwhelms me and I am driven into the ground with despair."
"I am exhausted, beaten to a pulp."
"I truly believe my headaches won't stop until I'm dead."

A brief history

References to headache date back 10,000 years. Primitive man thought head pain was caused by evil spirits invading the body and believed that the spirits had to be cut out. Using a trephine (a small crown saw), medicine men chiseled holes in the temples of the sufferers. Skulls with these types of bore markings dating back to the Neolithic and Bronze Ages have been found in Europe, Mexico, and Peru.

This procedure apparently brought some relief. Many skulls found in Europe display oval openings with edges that appear to be partly healed, indicating the surprising finding that the patients had survived their surgeries for some time.

The first written mention of headache is in the *Atharvaveda of India*, a treatise on magic formulas recorded between 1500 and 800 B.C.

The scientific age of medicine began with Hippocrates, the father of medicine, who was born on the island of Cos in 460 B.C. In his writings, he described the pain of a patient suffering from what was probably classic migraine (migraine with aura):

> *Most of the time he seemed to see something shining before him like a light, usually in part of the right eye; at the end of a moment, a violent pain supervened in the right temple, then in all the head and neck … vomiting, when it became possible, was able to divert the pain and render it more moderate.*

Aretaeus, a physician who practiced in Alexandria in 81 A.D., was the first to document the difference between migraine and a regular headache. He recognized that the pain was one-sided and that nausea was associated with the pain. He called the pain "heterocrania."

Galen, a Greek doctor who lived from 131 A.D. to 200 A.D., termed one-sided headache "hemicrania." This term is the source of the Old English word "megrim" and the French word "migraine."

Aurelius Cornelius Celsus (25 B.C. to 50 A.D.) was physician to the Roman emperors Tiberius and Caligula. He was the first to suggest that migraine is a nonfatal lifelong disorder with which trigger factors are associated. He also emphasized that the headache would be localized or generalized.

Over the years, many physicians tackled the causes and remedies of headaches. Thomas Willis (1621-1674), a London physician, wrote one of the first textbooks on the anatomy of the brain, *Cerebri Anatome*. The text, illustrated by Christopher Wren, the architect of St. Paul's Cathedral, divided headaches into those that were constant and those that were periodic, a distinction that remains of great importance today. Willis treated a female patient with "sick headache" for two decades and kept a diary of her suffering. Nothing he did seemed to work for her:

> *There was no kind of medicines, both cephalics, antiscor-buticks, hysterical, all forms specificks, which she took not,*

both from the learned and the unlearned, from quacks, and old women, and yet notwithstanding she professed that she had received from no remedy, or method of curing, any type of cure or ease, but that the contumacious and rebellious disease refused to be tamed, being deaf to the charms of every medicine.

The first significant book devoted only to headache was written by Edward Living in 1873 and titled *On Megrim, Sick Headache and Some Allied Disorders*, a contribution to the pathology of nerve storms. Though it had a very basic text, it was a milestone in recognizing headache as a primary medical disorder.

In 1948, Harold Wolff wrote *Headache and Other Pain*, the first comprehensive medical textbook on headache and specifically on migraine. It has been revised and updated over the years, but it is still considered the bible among headache books for physicians.

The biggest change in the understanding of migraine to arise since Wolff's work came about forty years later with the theory that migraine is primarily a brain or neurological condition with secondary, not primary, involvement of the vessels. The International Headache Society developed classification and diagnostic criteria for headaches in 1988. A revised version of this very long and detailed classification was published in 2005.

Basically headaches are classified as primary headaches (migraine, cluster, and tension-type) or secondary headaches (those headaches due to another disease or condition).

Another simplified classification is to divide headaches into those with a vascular component (migraine and cluster), tension headaches, and those due to traction or inflammation (secondary to other diseases).

Many neurologists consider the biggest breakthrough in headache medicine to be the development of the triptan drugs, particularly Imitrex, in the early 1990s. This was the first specific drug actually developed for migraine since the 1960s, when methysergide (Sansert) – a drug no longer available in the United States – was released.

"Magic" remedies

Sufferers have long been looking for a magic bullet, the one sure remedy that will end their pain. From the time of the Talmud – the book of Jewish law created between the 2nd and the 6th centuries – through the Middle Ages, the Renaissance, and into the 17th century, some of the more desperate remedies on record have included:

- Eating cashews
- Eating African ginger
- Wearing a crown woven of mugwort and wormwood

- Boiling a swallow's nest in water and applying it to the forehead
- Ingesting the herb valerian
- Applying roses and candied sugar to the head
- Applying a hot iron to the forehead
- Applying garlic to the forehead
- Using prayer or incantations
- Rubbing wine, oil, and vinegar on the head
- Drinking beer fortified with an onion crushed in honey
- Applying boiled frankincense, cumin, ulan berry, and Goose grease to the head
- Applying boiled torpedo fish to the head

Questionable cure-alls

In light of these previous therapeutic approaches, perhaps some of today's cure-alls don't seem so odd. Drugstore shelves and online websites are full of cures offering "fast relief" – not boiled torpedo fish or crowns of mugwort and wormwood, but plenty of products such as Head On (a homeopathic roll-on applied to the head), pills such as the Christian Body Migraine Defense, Sinus Buster (a natural pepper spray), Headache Relief Massager (battery-operated headgear with air chambers that inflate and deflate at the temples), and a variety of herbal remedies such as MigraEze ("guaranteed" by its makers to be a "breakthrough" product).

While some of these products contain ingredients that have been associated with headache relief, none of them is "guaranteed" to stop a headache.

Prosecutors recently asked a judge to halt the sale of products that allegedly were falsely advertised online by Flu Fighters Laboratories Inc., a company in Boca Raton, Florida. The company was peddling several products, including a migraine remedy called Migraine Miracle that Flu Fighters claimed was approved by the Food and Drug Administration. It was not.

Famous headache sufferers

General Ulysses S. Grant, Sigmund Freud, and Charles Darwin all suffered with migraines and recorded their miseries in diaries and journals.

Many authors – among them Mark Twain, George Bernard Shaw, Rudyard Kipling, Ralph Waldo Emerson, Emily Dickinson, William Shakespeare, Lewis Carroll, John Steinbeck, Joan Didion, and Stephen King – have made reference to migraines in the pages of their books.

Ulysses S. Grant

Charles Darwin

Mark Twain

Steinbeck may have been a headache sufferer – or was certainly around someone who was – because he was easily able to describe the migraine suffering of Mrs. Pritchard in his 1947 book *The Wayward Bus*:

> *Her husband knew her headaches, and they were dreadful. They twisted her face and reduced her to a panting, sweating, grinning, quivering blob of pain. They filled a room and a house. They got into everyone around her.*

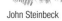
John Steinbeck

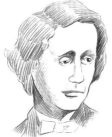
Lewis Carroll

Author Lewis Carroll reportedly suffered from migraine attacks. In his journal he called them "bilious headaches." It is believed that several passages in *Alice in Wonderland* describe his experiences with migraine aura (sensory phenomena that may occur before a migraine). When Alice drank the bottle marked "Drink Me" and began to shrink, Carroll seemed to be referring to a type of migraine aura in which a sufferer's body image is altered. Later, Alice ate a cake marked "Eat Me" and began to grow. Patients who suffer with this type of aura are said to have the "Alice in Wonderland" syndrome.

George Bernard Shaw

Tweedledum, one of Carroll's fictional twins, also had headache problems. He explained one day, "I'm very brave generally. Only today I have a headache."

Chronic headaches can make a wimp out of the bravest soul. Headaches are a legitimate biological disease. Migraine is a disorder just as real as hypertension or diabetes. For today's headache sufferers, once a correct diagnosis is made, an effective treatment plan can be started. Headache specialists know how to dramatically reduce headache frequency and severity through a combination of drug and non-drug therapies.

William Shakespeare

Rudyard Kipling

Ralph Waldo Emerson

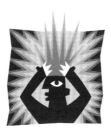

Chapter 2

Tension-type Headaches

Photojournalist Kathleen Smith works from 10 a.m. to 7 p.m. at a large metropolitan newspaper in South Florida. By midafternoon, she has traveled to several assignments and photographed a children's play, the return of a Major League baseball team to spring-training camp, and a ten-car pileup on Interstate-95.

Having worked through her lunch hour, she feels her head begin to pound. Her editor, in touch on the two-way radio, urges her to hurry back to the office. While rushing to meet her deadline, she finds herself stuck in a traffic jam, with no movement for miles. Now her head is really pounding.

Fumbling through her purse, she grabs her huge, trusty bottle of acetaminophen and pops two pills, washing them down with a day-old bottle of lemonade. Her job is a demanding one and, day after day, she finds herself reaching for her headache pills.

Tension-type headache, often referred to as "stress" headache, is the most common headache type, yet we know very little about it because migraine and cluster headaches receive much more attention, research, and investigation.

Nearly 200 million people in the United States suffer from tension-type headache. Tension-type headache is usually episodic, but it may be considered chronic if it occurs daily or almost daily for more than fifteen days a month. Women between the ages of 30 and 50 are most likely to experience chronic tension-type headaches.

The headaches can be of mild to moderate intensity, with a constant bandlike pain coupled with pressure or throbbing that affects the front, top, or sides of the head. The neck often feels tight and stiff. The discomfort level is usually mild to moderate and does not worsen with activity.

The International Headache Society distinguishes between three categories of tension-type headaches:

- **Episodic.** This headache occurs less than once a month and the pain is mild to moderate.
- **Frequent.** This occurs fewer than fifteen days per month. The pain is mild to moderate, with constant bandlike pressure or throbbing on the top, front, and sides of the head. It can last thirty minutes to several days.
- **Chronic.** This occurs more than fifteen days a month. The pain is always present and varies in intensity, affect-

ing the front, sides, and top of the head, and it comes and goes over a long period of time.

Although the chronic variety of this type of headache occurs in only slightly more than 2 percent of the population, it accounts for many missed workdays and plenty of visits to the doctor's office.

Daily headache may occur as a chronic tension-type headache, but it is often a combination of tension-type and migraine. This type of combination headache is not listed in the official classification, so a doctor will often diagnose both chronic tension-type headache and migraine. Most often, this type of "mixed" headache arises in an individual who initially had typical episodic migraine but over the years develops a daily or near-daily headache. Many times the daily headache is a consequence of the overuse of analgesics, barbiturates, ergotamine tartrate (a drug that constricts blood vessels), or any of the triptan drugs that are used to treat migraines. This headache pattern is called **rebound headache** or **medication-overuse headache**.

Each of these three categories of tension-type headache is further broken down by whether there is evidence of tenderness of the pericranium muscle (the dense tissue covering the skull).

Tension-type headache attributed to increased pericranial muscle tension is often due to neck injury such as whiplash, poor posture with slouching or rounded shoulders, or temporomandibular joint disorders such as clenching or grinding of the teeth.

Individuals who show evidence of muscle tenderness and increased muscle contraction or spasm often benefit from muscle relaxants, physical therapy (such as heat, exercise, and massage), and tender-point or trigger-point injections of cortisone and a local anesthetic.

Whether there's increased muscle contraction or not, the discomfort described is usually the same. Several studies have shown that people who suffer from this type of headache often are dealing with depression, anxiety, or suppressed anger. Other common symptoms of headache sufferers are difficulty sleeping, inability to concentrate, irritability, and chronic fatigue. Although nausea and sensitivity to light and sound may occur, generally they are not prominent features. These headaches are generally not as debilitating as migraine or cluster headaches.

No one knows what causes tension headache, but stress, fatigue, depression, anxiety, and emotional conflicts are thought to contribute. Headaches often occur in the middle of the day, beginning gradually and lasting anywhere from half an hour to several days. There are no dietary triggers for tension headache.

The occasional tension-type headache can be alleviated by a hot shower, massage, and sleep, and by avoiding stressors. Usually, episodic tension-type headache is easily treated with analgesics such as aspirin, acetaminophen, and the NSAIDs (nonsteroidal anti-inflammatory drugs that decrease swelling and pain), or combinations of these agents with caffeine or sedative medications. Some patients, particularly those with tension-type headache caused by stress, may benefit from relaxation techniques or biofeedback training. Physical therapy may also decrease chronic neck pain caused by increased cervical muscle spasm or bad posture, which may place undue stress on certain areas of the body.

When tension-type headache becomes chronic, treatment can be challenging, especially if the patient overuses analgesics and opiates. Treatment will not be effective until the patient stops taking these acute pain-relieving agents on a daily basis. Often, patients suffering from chronic tension-type headache need counseling and psychotherapy to help define and work through long-standing psychological issues.

 The most effective group of drugs for treatment of chronic tension-type headaches is that of the tricyclic antidepressants, the most common of which are amitriptyline HCl (Elavil), doxepin HCl (Sinequan), and nortriptyline HCl (Pamelor). Because of their sedating effects, they are usually taken at bedtime. Morning sedation, weight gain, dry mouth, and constipation are common side effects.

Less sedating drugs in this group are desipramine HCl (Norpramin) and protriptyline HCl (Vivactil). Serotonin reuptake inhibitors such as fluoxetine HCl (Prozac), sertraline HCl

(Zoloft), paroxetine HCl (Paxil), and citalopram hydrobromide (Celexa) are better tolerated and have fewer side effects than the tricyclics, but they do not appear to be as effective in easing headache unless the headache is a manifestation of underlying depression. Venlafaxine HCl (Effexor) and duloxetine HCl (Cymbalta) are both serotonin and norepinephrine uptake inhibitors and may be helpful in chronic pain conditions, including headache. Muscle relaxants such as cyclobenzaprine HCl (Flexeril), orphenadrine citrate (Norflex), methocarbamol (Robaxin), and baclofen (Lioresal) may be helpful at times, particularly if increased muscle spasm is present. Carisoprodol (Soma), a muscle relaxant, should not be used for any extended period of time because it can produce dependency.

In recent clinical trials, the central-acting muscle relaxant tizanidine HCl (Zanaflex) was found to be effective in treating chronic headache, whether tension-type or coexisting migraine and tension-type.

Treatment approaches

Ten years ago, when Doug DeMeter bought his own car dealership, the headaches began. "It coincided with the computer age for me," says Doug. He'd spend hours each day staring into his computer and worrying about things he couldn't control. Sometimes a couple of cups of coffee each morning would knock out the pain.

He was constantly taking aspirin. Doug began to worry that something might be really wrong.

As a kid, he had played a number of sports and had sustained several concussions. "I was the little guy, so I got beat up a lot," he remembers. He wondered whether these new headaches might have something to do with his feisty youth.

After seeing his doctor, he had a CAT scan. The scan was perfectly normal – which was the good news. But what could he do to stop his horrible headaches?

Trying to figure out possible underlying causes of headache may alter the approach to treatment.

The first line of defense is a nonprescription analgesic such as aspirin, acetaminophen, or ibuprofen. However, using a daily analgesic can cause rebound headache. An occasional headache becomes a daily headache, and the medication that used to work no longer does the job.

Caffeine can sometimes stop a headache cold. Studies of a drug containing ibuprofen and caffeine have shown some promise, but the drug is not available in the United States. Unfortunately, the frequent use of caffeine can also cause rebound headache.

As mentioned earlier, the antidepressant drugs are the most effective agents in treating chronic tension-type headaches. These drugs are good choices for chronic tension-type headache that may or may not accompany depression. The dosage needed to relieve pain is at a lower level than that which is needed to treat depression.

If there is tenderness and tightness or spasm of the neck and scalp muscles, muscle relaxants such as Zanaflex (tizanidine) or Flexeril (cyclobenzaprine) may also be prescribed.

Lifestyle changes can go a long way toward easing headache pain. It's important to eat a balanced diet, get plenty of sleep, and exercise regularly. Such approaches as physical therapy, massage, acupuncture, stress management, relaxation training, biofeedback, or meditation may help. If depression is a problem, psychological counseling may be recommended. (See Chapter 6: "Alternatives.")

For Kathleen and Doug, lifestyle changes, stress reduction, and a low dose of the tricyclic antidepressant Elavil (amitriptyline) worked wonders. Both have been on the drug for a decade. "It changed my life," says Doug.

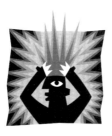

Chapter 3

Migraines

When Suzanne Harris shows up for work in the morning, she frequently has an ice bag strapped to her head. No one bats an eye – her co-workers are used to it. At least she shows up.

Diagnosed with migraines at the age of 34, Suzanne, now 50, is a frequent migraine sufferer and has tried just about everything to alleviate the constant, pounding ache behind her left eye. Like most headache sufferers, she has her own routines that she practices when migraines attack. She'll try whatever it takes to lessen the pain. The ice bag provides relief so she wears it.

Over the years, her headache doctors have placed her on a variety of medications in an attempt to find just the right drug. She has tried antidepressants, anticonvulsants, and beta-blockers with some relief, though many of them caused unpleasant side effects. For Suzanne, now getting relief from one of the newer triptan drugs, finding the right medication has been a long, exhausting process.

Sue Jacobs, 35, was sitting at her office computer when she first saw little white spots floating before her eyes. She blinked, thinking perhaps it was time to visit the eye doctor for a new prescription. Before long, the white spots merged completely, blocking her vision for more than thirty minutes. "There was no pain," says Sue. "I really didn't think of it as a headache."

Her ophthalmologist found nothing wrong with her vision but diagnosed her right away: aura **without** *migraine headache, a condition that usually occurs later in life. Though some migraine sufferers get a similar sensation just before a painful migraine hits, Jacobs never felt any pain.*

Fifteen years later, Sue is coping with the reverse problem: painful migraines **without** *aura. She has no more white spots, but there's plenty of pain. She, too, has tried numerous medications and is finally finding relief with one of the triptan drugs.*

There is no cure for migraine. No magic bullet, all-purpose pill, or perfect treatment plan. For the longtime migraine sufferer, it seems incredible that the "trial-and-error" search for an effective medication is still part of the grueling process of learning to manage the pain.

But migraines can be managed, and health-care professionals are adding new treatments to their arsenals that can stop a migraine attack and prevent future attacks.

About fifteen years ago, the development of the triptan drugs (such as Imitrex) revolutionized the treatment of migraines and cluster headaches. As previously noted, it was the first specific drug actually developed for migraine since methysergide (Sansert) in the 1960s.

Inderal, a beta-blocker, became available for the treatment of hypertension in the early 1970s and was found to help prevent migraine as well. Since the early 1990s, more triptan drugs have been developed, and they are now the drugs of choice for treating mild, moderate, and severe migraine attacks in most sufferers. All the triptans (currently seven) are effective in about 70 percent of migraine patients.

However, a therapy that works for one person may not work for another. It is important for patients to be proactive, diligent, and willing to work with their doctors to find a treatment plan that works.

Who has migraines?

Twenty-eight million Americans suffer from migraines and about half of them don't even know it. Armed with bottles of over-the-counter medications, many folks take on the task of taming their headaches alone.

For instance, many people who think they're suffering from a "sinus headache" resulting from allergies or weather changes may pop a few pills and wait for the weather to change. While allergies do not cause migraines, they can cause nasal and sinus congestion, and headaches may be the result.

Research has shown that even if the headache is not severe enough to require bed rest and even when over-the-counter medications seem to provide some relief, many people who think they have recurring sinus headaches are actually suffering from migraine. And because they have never been properly diagnosed, they may not be taking the right steps to obtain relief. In fact, frequent use of over-the-counter medication may cause frequent, recurring headaches.

Overuse can lead to rebound headache, a dull, low-grade daily headache. The headache will respond to the overused medication but will recur in a few hours, necessitating another dose. Relief from this type of headache can only be accomplished by completely stopping all pain medications. This should be done under the supervision of a doctor.

Most migraine sufferers are women between the ages of 15 and 55. Migraine occurs about three times more often in women than men. Migraine is an inherited condition; more than 70 percent of people suffering from migraines have a family history of the disorder and may inherit the tendency to be affected by migraine triggers such as fatigue, bright lights, or weather changes. One in every four homes includes a migraine sufferer.

Though there is some debate among experts, it appears that migraine sufferers tend to be inflexible perfectionists who are inclined to take on more than they can handle. Scientists also believe that the inability to cope with anxiety, anger, and stress may cause the onset of a migraine. Diet, changing hormone levels, weather, altitude changes, and lifestyle factors also may contribute to migraine attacks.

The frequency of migraines varies widely among individuals. The average migraine sufferer gets two to four headaches each month. Some people may get headaches every few days, while others have a migraine only once or twice a year. Along with rebound headache (due to overuse of medication), chronic migraine (more than fifteen headache days a month) is the most common type of headache treated at headache clinics.

Asthma, hypertension, stroke, sleep disorders, chronic fatigue syndrome, fibromyalgia, and temporomandibular (TMJ) joint disorder are a few of the medical conditions that may be associated with migraines. Chronic daily headaches can also be associated with depression and anxiety.

No one is really sure what brain abnormality underlies migraine. For years, scientists thought that the main culprit was vascular instability – circumstances in which the blood vessels periodically constrict (narrow) and then dilate (expand). Now, the prevailing belief is that migraines are triggered within the brain.

Once the attack begins, the pain and other symptoms come from an inflammatory process resulting from an interaction between the trigeminal nerve (which originates in the brainstem) and blood vessels in the coverings of the brain and in the scalp.

It is thought that a migraine begins when hyperactive nerve cells in the brain send out impulses over the trigeminal nerve to blood vessels, causing them to constrict. This is followed by dilation of the vessels and the release of prostaglandins, serotonin, and several other inflammatory substances into the surrounding tissue. This inflammation causes the pulsation in the vessels to become painful.

Pain signals are then carried back from the inflamed blood vessels along the trigeminal nerve into the brain. The pain-processing centers in the brainstem then become overloaded by the incoming pain signals and begin to fire off more impulses, causing a self-perpetuating condition.

While migraine headache usually affects only one side of the head, it may involve the entire head. It may last for several hours or even days.

Trigeminal nerve

Pia mater ⎤
Arachnoid ⎬ Meninges
Dura mater ⎦

Skull

Blood vessel

Types of migraine

There are two basic types of migraine:

- **With aura** (also known as "classic" migraine)
- **Without aura** (also known as "common" migraine)

There are four phases to a migraine attack:

- **Prodrome**. This can occur days or hours before an attack. The sufferer may experience food cravings, fatigue, mood changes, and extreme sensitivity to light or sounds.
- **Aura**. Only about 20 percent of migraine sufferers experience an aura, which is usually a visual warning sign that a migraine is about to begin. These symptoms usually occur thirty to sixty minutes before the onset of an acute migraine attack and may include light flashes, blind spots, or geometric patterns that obscure vision. Other senses may also be affected: Unusual sounds or smells may be experienced. Some people may experience an aura with tingling or numbing sensations in the arm and face prior to the head pain. Occasionally, a neurological aura will occur, causing a tingling or weakness that slowly spreads up or down an extremity. The warning symptoms clear as the pain begins. Sometimes a migraine aura may occur without a headache; this phenomenon tends to occur in later in life, but it can occur anytime.

- **Headache.** This is a throbbing head pain, usually on one side of the head. The pain is aggravated by any physical activity. Sensitivity to sound and light is very common. Nausea occurs in most patients and vomiting is common, as is sensitivity to odors, dizziness, and diarrhea. Dehydration may occur, which will increase the pain and disability of the condition. Sufferers want to remain quiet and inactive in a darkened area during the attack, which can last from four to seventy-two hours.
- **Postdrome.** This is the "migraine hangover." Most patients feel exhausted, weak, and irritable. However, some patients may also experience sensations of unusual joy and exhilaration.

Treatment plans are based on headache history, frequency of attacks, degree of disability, and several other factors. Migraine sufferers are encouraged to track the episodes in a headache diary to assist their health-care professionals in learning more about their symptoms. Recording when the migraine begins, how long it lasts, possible triggers, and a detailed description of the pain will help doctors form a treatment plan that will work.

Medications

Two types of medication are recommended for patients suffering from migraines:

- **Preventive.** For patients who suffer more than two migraine attacks per month, these medications are taken on a daily basis and can reduce the number and severity of attacks. They are not effective if taken after a migraine begins, so it is important for the patient to have a symptomatic medication available as well to stop the attack. These preventive medications are usually available only by prescription and include beta-blockers such as propranolol (Inderal), nadolol (Corgard), atenolol (Tenormin), metoprolol (Toprol, Lopresser), and timolol (Blocadren); calcium-channel blockers such as verapamil (Calan, Isoptin); antidepressants such as amitriptyline (Elavil), nortriptyline (Pamelor), fluoxetine (Prozac), venlafaxine (Effexor), and duloxetine (Cymbalta); antiseizure medications such as divalproex sodium (Depakote), gabapentin (Neurontin), topiramate (Topamax), or pregabalin (Lyrica); and nonsteroidal anti-inflammatory drugs (NSAIDs). Some of these drugs may require a trial of a few months to become effective. Antidepressants and tranquilizers used to treat anxiety can also be very effective in the treatment of some migraines.

- **Abortive.** All patients, whether they're on preventive medication or not, will need something for the acute attacks. Abortive medications relieve the pain and symptoms once an attack has begun. These medications work best if taken very early in the attack. Some of these medications include ergotamine tartrate in combination with caffeine (Cafergot), dihydroergotamine (Migranal, DHE 45), and isometheptene (Midrin). The triptans, the newest highly successful drugs, include almotriptan (Axert), frovatriptan (Frova), naratriptan (Amerge), rizatriptan (Maxalt), sumatriptan (Imitrex), zolmitriptan (Zomig), and eletriptan (Relpax). These drugs should not be used by patients with a history of stroke, heart attack, or serious hypertension.

Triptan drugs significantly relieve migraine pain and associated symptoms within two hours of administration. The earlier in the attack that they are taken, the more effective they seem to be. Headache recurs within twenty-four hours in up to 30 percent of users, necessitating an additional dose. All these triptan drugs are effective in about 70 percent of persons with migraine. Use of an NSAID in combination with a triptan may offer better headache relief and less frequent recurrence.

At times, a rescue medication such as an opiate or butalbital combination drug may be needed, but with the large number of non-habit-forming preparations available, there is less need for such a drug. Some oral abortive agents, especially the ergotamines, often cause nausea and vomiting, but patients using an antiemetic drug such as metoclopramide before they take the ergotamine may be able to control the nausea and also enhance the effectiveness of the abortive drug.

Some over-the-counter drugs are effective in treating migraines. The FDA has approved Excedrin Migraine, a combination of aspirin, acetaminophen, and caffeine, and Advil Migraine and Motrin Migraine Pain (two ibuprofen products) for relief of mild or moderate migraine.

Cleveland Clinic's Headache Clinic has been a pioneer in the development of an "infusion center." Clinic patients who have urgent headache needs or headaches that have not responded to treatment at home may visit the center and receive non-narcotic intravenous treatments that traditionally would have required a trip to an emergency room or perhaps even hospitalization.

Such comprehensive outpatient-treatment programs are now being used by many headache clinics, and many of the patients treated are suffering from chronic daily headaches and medication overuse. Most programs include detoxification from analgesics and narcotics, the initiation of preventive medicines, psychotherapy, physical therapy, the teaching of relaxation and biofeedback techniques, and educating patients to become aware of and recognize triggers that may set off their headaches.

Status migrainosus

Status migrainosus is the term used for a migraine attack that lasts longer than seventy-two hours. It can be a migraine that doesn't respond to acute abortive medication or one that did respond but keeps recurring after treatment with triptans, ergotamine, or analgesics.

Since we now know that the triptans or other abortive medications work much better when taken very early in the attack, it's essential that patients learn to recognize when a migraine is developing and take their medication as early as possible. Doing this will increase the likelihood of a response and decrease the likelihood of getting into a non-responding or recurring headache that will become a status migraine.

Probably the main reason why early treatment is more effective is that one needs to stop the headache before the neurons become sensitized as the headache progresses. When neurons in the brain become less responsive to medications and more sensitized, sufferers develop cutaneous allodynia (the scalp becomes painful to touch or stimulation). Another reason that early treatment is more effective is that the digestive system shuts down if nausea and vomiting develop. Once nausea develops, it's very hard for the digestive system to absorb oral medication.

A main concern with a prolonged migraine attack is that the sufferer will continue to use abortive medications or pain medications in an effort to break the attack and then may get into "rebounding" – the return of the headache's original symptoms.

No one knows how long it takes for the daily use of analgesics, caffeine, ergotamines, or triptans to cause one to develop a rebound headache. In some people, this may occur after a short time. However, most researchers in the headache field feel that it takes weeks or months of daily use before one gets into a true rebounding or "medication overuse" state.

Giving patients who are experiencing a prolonged migraine several doses of cortisone usually breaks the siege. But this may not be feasible if the patient is vomiting. The use of a cortisone drug is limited to no more than once a month to avoid any long-term side effects, which may include decreased bone density, easy bruising, ulcer disease, and high blood pressure. However, many people, after a few days of nonstop migraine, will head for the emergency room or a doctor's office to get a shot. The shot given is often a narcotic and a sedative. Studies show that this type of treatment rarely stops the headache but does cause some relief of the severe pain and often produces sleep. Many patients have been vomiting and have become dehydrated, which aggravates the headache.

Sleep, of course, is one of the best treatments for a migraine attack. So if the pain can be relieved enough to allow sleep or a sedating drug to promote sleep is given, the headache will often break.

Basilar migraine

Basilar migraine is a rare form of migraine with aura. The aura, which usually lasts about an hour, may be associated with visual symptoms on both sides of the head, dizziness (often vertigo with a spinning sensation), balance problems, bilateral numbness, nausea, speech disturbances, and temporary blindness. After the aura passes, it is usually followed by a typical migraine headache. This type of migraine most commonly affects young adults.

Symptoms come from disturbances in the brainstem or both sides of the brain. Because of the dizziness and slurred speech, sufferers may appear intoxicated by drugs or alcohol.

Hemiplegic migraine

Hemiplegic migraine (whereby sufferers experience numbness, weakness, or paralysis of one side of the body) affects a very small segment of the population. Attacks can begin in childhood, adolescence, or during early adulthood, but are uncommon in people over 50 years of age.

Hemiplegic attacks are accompanied by aura and often feature visual disturbances and speech difficulty. Sometimes sufferers may be diagnosed as experiencing a stroke, epilepsy, or multiple sclerosis.

When this type of migraine runs in families, it is called *familial hemiplegic migraine*. It occurs in several generations, with all sufferers having the same neurological symptoms. Sufferers who do not have other family members with similar problems are said to have *sporadic hemiplegic migraine*.

Recently, genetic research has found three different genetic defects that can cause familial hemiplegic migraine, and genetic testing for these abnormalities is now available in the United States.

The triptan medications so useful to most migraine sufferers are *not* advised here. Verapamil (a calcium-channel blocker) and the antiepileptic drugs may be helpful in decreasing the severity and frequency of hemiplegic migraine attacks.

Menstrual migraines

"Menstrual migraine" and "menstrual-related migraine" are confusing terms.

Many women develop migraine in their teens around the onset of menstruation. The term "menstrual migraine" refers to a migraine headache that occurs *only* within the two days before or the two days after the onset of the menstrual flow and does not occur at any other time of the month.

This pattern is not very common. However, more than 60 percent of women with migraine have "menstrual-related migraine." Their worst migraine attacks occur in association with the menstrual period, but they also experience migraine attacks at other times. This type of migraine may become more common as women reach their 40s and perimenopause (the years just prior to menopause), and there may be worsening of migraines as a result of irregular cycles that make migraine attacks less predictable. After women reach menopause, attacks tend to subside.

During ovulation and menstruation, fluctuating levels of estrogen and progesterone can trigger migraine. Sixty percent of women who suffer from migraine report an increase in the frequency and severity of headaches during their menstrual period (menstrual related migraine), while 10 to 15 percent say their headaches occur only at this time (menstrual migraine). Of these women, 60 percent to 70 percent report their worst attacks during the period of premenstrual flow.

Estrogen levels drop immediately before the start of the menstrual flow, and premenstrual migraines usually occur during or after the time when the female hormones – estrogen and progesterone – are at their lowest levels.

Hormone-replacement therapy can have a positive effect on migraines. Many women with bad menstrual migraines are now being given oral contraceptives daily for a three-month cycle, rather than for a one-month cycle, which reduces the frequency of severe attacks. Though added estrogen can trigger and worsen migraines in some women, 45 percent say that the therapy reduces the number of headaches they get.

Triggers

Migraine triggers differ from person to person. Diet, activity, environment, emotions, medications, and hormones are some main triggers. Identifying triggers requires a fair bit of detective work by the patient, but avoiding these triggers will result in fewer headaches.

The most common food, beverages, and additives that may trigger headache pain are:

- **Smoking.** Nicotine stimulates constriction of the blood vessels in the brain. It also stimulates nerves in the back of the throat that may contribute to headache pain.
- **Alcohol.** Blood flow to the brain increases when you drink. Watch out for red wine, beer, whiskey, and champagne.
- **Aged cheeses and other foods containing tyramine.** Tyramine is a naturally occurring substance found in some foods and is formed from the breakdown of protein as food ages. It is also found in red wine, alcoholic beverages, and some processed meats.
- **Food additives.** Preservatives such as nitrates dilate blood vessels, causing headaches in some people. Monosodium glutamate (MSG), a flavor enhancer added to many prepared foods, may also trigger migraine.
- **Cold foods.** Icy drinks or ice cream can cause headaches, especially if you're overheated. This type of pain, some-

times called "brain freeze," can last from several seconds to several minutes.

- **Caffeine.** Caffeine is both a headache treatment and a headache trigger. It is commonly found in many over-the-counter headache medications. It can make the medication 40 percent more effective by helping the body absorb it more quickly. However, the daily use of medication containing caffeine and consumption of too much caffeine from coffee, tea, chocolate, or soft drinks can sensitize the blood vessels so that when caffeine is not ingested, a withdrawal-type of headache (rebound headache) may occur.

Other common migraine triggers are:

- **Emotional stress.** During stress, chemicals in the brain are released to combat the situation (known as "fight-or-flight response"). Anxiety, worry, excitement, and fatigue can increase muscle tension, and dilated blood vessels can intensify the severity of the migraine.
- **Changing weather conditions.** Changes in barometric pressure, altitude, and strong winds or weather fronts can trigger a migraine. Some sufferers do a fairly good job of managing their headaches by paying attention to the weather and staying ahead of the forecast.
- **Excessive fatigue.**

- Skipping meals.
- Changes in normal sleep patterns.

About 30 percent of migraine sufferers are able to link some of their headaches to specific dietary triggers. Foods that may trigger headaches include:

- Peanuts, peanut butter, other nuts, and seeds
- Pizza
- Potato chips
- Chicken livers and other organ meats
- Smoked or dried fish
- Crackers, freshly baked products such as donuts and cakes, and baked goods containing yeast, such as homemade rolls, sourdough bread, and other breads
- Desserts containing cheese
- Certain fresh fruits, including ripe bananas, citrus fruits, papaya, red plums, raspberries, kiwi, and pineapple
- Dried fruits
- Soups made from meat extracts or bouillon
- Cultured dairy products such as sour cream, yogurt, or buttermilk
- Aspartame and other artificial sweeteners

Headaches from food additives usually begin within twenty to thirty minutes of consumption. Pressure in the chest and face; a burning sensation in the chest, neck, or shoulders; facial flushing; dizziness; and abdominal pain may occur.

Also, be careful of food additives in the following:

- Hot dogs
- Ham
- Sausage
- Bacon
- Luncheon meats and deli-style meats
- Pepperoni
- Other cured or processed meats
- Some heart medications
- MSG, the additive/flavor-enhancer found in food served at some Chinese restaurants as well as in soy sauce, meat tenderizer, Asian foods, and many packaged foods

How you can help yourself

Getting a proper diagnosis is key. It can mean more than just stopping the crippling pain: Migraine headaches have been linked to some serious conditions, including stroke and obesity. The average risk of stroke for all migraine sufferers is about 2.16 times more than that of those who do not suffer from migraine. And migraine sufferers who take oral contraceptives may have an eight times greater risk for stroke, since changes in blood flow to the brain during an attack can cause dangerous clotting. The estrogens may also make women more prone to developing blood clots. The increased risk seems to be more likely in those suffering migraine with aura.

Some studies suggest that women who have migraine with aura may have an increased risk of heart disease. A recent study at Brigham and Women's Hospital and the Harvard School of Public Health in Boston found that women age 45 and older who suffer from migraine with aura have a slightly higher risk for angina, heart attack, ischemic stroke, and death than do women who experience no migraines.

Be proactive. Take control of your health by:

- Supplying your health-care provider with a list of all the medications you're taking.
- Knowing your headache history. During your doctor's evaluation, be prepared to answer questions about your family history, the age at which you began having attacks, their frequency, and their duration.
- Being able to describe your symptoms and migraine attacks with as much information as possible. If you have been treated in the past for headache or have copies of your imaging tests, make them available, and bring a list of your previous medications.

Tests

Your doctor should perform a complete physical and neurological examination. Headache can be the first symptom of a much worse illness such as brain tumor, cerebral hemorrhage, epilepsy, or multiple sclerosis. Fortunately, this is usually not the case – less than 2 percent of all headaches are caused by an underlying disease. The examination and tests focus on ruling out these problems, yet they can also identify a structural abnormality in the brain that may be causing your headaches.

The following tests may be recommended:

- **Magnetic resonance imaging (MRI)**. This test provides information about the structure and biochemistry of the brain.
- **Computed axial tomography (CT scan)**. This test uses x-rays and computers to produce an image of a cross-section of areas of the body.

Sometimes your doctor may recommend an interview with a psychologist in order to identify stress factors that may be triggering your headaches. Maintaining regular schedules for sleeping, eating, and exercising has been shown to cut the number of attacks.

Non-drug treatments such as relaxation techniques, exercise, biofeedback, acupuncture, and massage can be effective when used along with medication. (See Chapter 6, "Alternatives.")

Hole in the heart/patent foramen ovale

Can migraine be treated with outpatient heart surgery? Many patients with migraine are asking for an evaluation of whether they have "a hole in the heart." Over the last few years, several reports have suggested that closure of a patent foramen ovale has been associated with reduced frequency and severity of migraine with aura. However, closure of this defect does not seem to have a significant benefit on migraine without aura.

The foramen ovale is an opening in the septum that separates the left and right upper chambers (atria) of the heart. This hole is present in the heart of the developing fetus to allow circulating blood to bypass the lungs, since the lungs are not used for oxygenating the blood. After birth, the foramen ovale usually closes; however, about 25 percent of the time, it does not close completely. Usually, this doesn't cause any problems and doesn't affect the functioning of the heart.

The initial reports of benefit in migraine were from persons who had migraine and had suffered a stroke. During an exam searching for possible causes of the stroke, if a patent (open) foramen ovale was found, it was patched and closed. After the closure, many people then reported less frequent and less severe migraine attacks. In analyzing these reports, the improvement was almost always in those who suffered from migraine with aura.

Determination of the presence of a hole can be made with an echocardiogram and other cardiac tests. A closure patch can then be placed over the defect by means of a catheter in the veins – a procedure similar to a heart catheterization.

It is uncertain how patching a hole is associated with a decrease in migraine with aura. One theory holds that certain chemical substances (perhaps hormonal in nature), which circulate in the blood and are usually removed as the blood passes through the lungs, may reach the brain by passing through the hole, triggering a migraine attack.

Studies are being conducted in which some migraine sufferers will receive patches and others will have a catheter inserted but will not be patched. Hopefully, the research will prove whether patching the hole has a real effect on migraine with aura or whether the reported improvement is merely a "placebo effect." Over the years, many surgical procedures have been performed that attempted to control migraine, but none has stood the test of time.

The cover image and the illustrations on the following pages were among the winners in "Migraine Masterpieces: My Life with Migraine," an art contest for migraine sufferers sponsored by the National Headache Foundation. They are used with permission. For more information on headache causes and treatments, visit www.headaches.org.

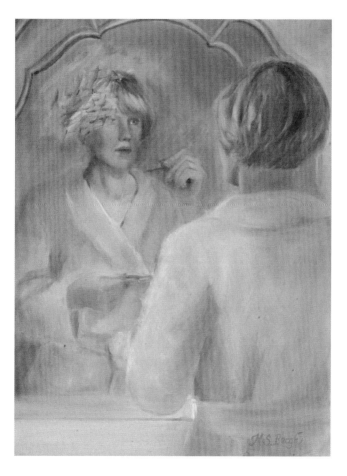

"Scotoma, the Abyssal Pain," by Maxine Bergh.

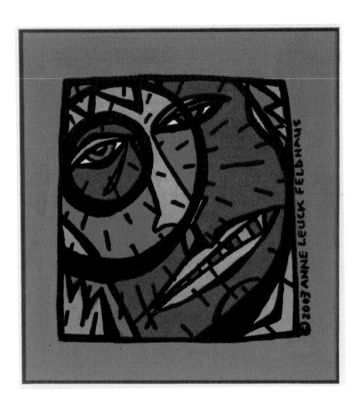

"Bull's Eye," by Anne Feldhaus.

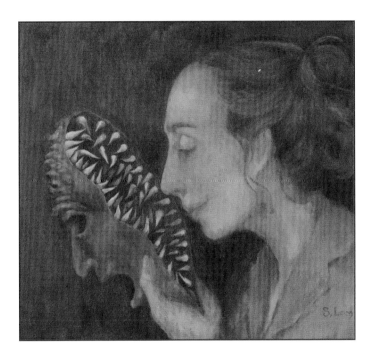

"Taking Off the Migraine Mask," by Sarah Leon.

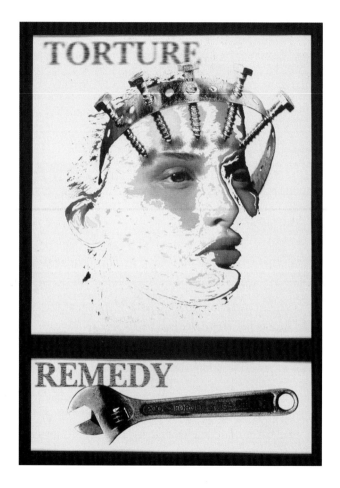

"Torture/Remedy #2," by Jean Thomas.

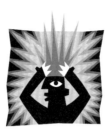

Chapter 4

Cluster Headaches

David Marshall, 56, dreads bedtime. A classic longtime cluster-headache sufferer, David knows when he climbs into bed every evening that there's a good possibility he'll awaken at exactly 1:30 a.m. with an excruciating pain behind his left eye. "There are nights I don't want to go to sleep," says David. "I'm afraid."

For David this fear has been haunting him for twenty-five years, nearly half his life. When he was a younger man, David used to pace the house, threatening to bang his head against the stone fireplace in his basement. He'd try anything to stop the constant burning pain. Like a hot poker jabbed into his left eye, the pain continued across his forehead and down the side of his temple into his ear. "The real bad ones go down my neck and into the jaw," he says. "Even my teeth hurt."

Cluster headache, also known as Horton's headache, hista-mine headache, or "alarm-clock" or "suicide" headache, is the most severe and least common type of the primary headaches. It can be 100 times more intense than a migraine. The pain has caused patients to attempt suicide – some have actually committed the act – during an acute attack. The reference to alarm clocks refers to the fact that the patient's headaches often occur at the same time each day during the cycle, frequently in the middle of the night, and often wake the patient in the early morning hours.

There are two types of cluster headaches:

- **Episodic.** This type is the most common. The headaches appear in periods or clusters lasting from seven days up to one year and are separated by headache-free intervals that last at least two weeks. The period of attacks usually lasts from two weeks to three months and recurs within six months to a year. Some people will go two to three years between clusters, while others may have two to three bouts of headaches in a year.
- **Chronic.** This type is long-term with no significant break. The headaches occur for more than one year with no remission or with remissions that last less than two weeks. Perhaps 10 percent of cluster sufferers will have one of these prolonged sieges.

The pain of cluster is constant and piercing, and usually located behind one eye. It comes on suddenly and with a vengeance. The pain usually peaks in a few minutes, but will last twenty minutes to four hours and may be so intense that sufferers will pace the floor, bang their head on the wall, or do vigorous exercises during the attack.

About 80 percent of sufferers experience nasal congestion and a teary, reddened eye on the side where the pain occurs. Twenty percent will have drooping of the eyelid on the affected side. Nausea and vomiting, so common in migraine, rarely occur in cluster. These symptoms clear as the headache eases. The headache disappears but may recur later in the day. Cluster attacks usually occur one to three times a day during a cluster period that may last two weeks to three months. Attacks seem to occur more frequently in spring and fall, and are often mistakenly associated with allergies and sinus.

Cluster headaches are not caused by serious underlying conditions such as an aneurysm or tumor. No one knows what causes cluster headaches, but many experts believe that this disorder involves a part of the brain called the hypothalamus, the brain's internal biological clock. It is thought that for some reason nerve cells in this area periodically become sensitized and begin firing impulses over the trigeminal nerve, which activates sensations to the head, brain, and face. This causes eye pain and stimulates another group of nerves that cause nasal congestion and teary, red eyes. There is also a marked increase in the blood flow through the internal carotid artery on the headache side during the attack of pain, due to a marked dilation (opening up) of the blood vessels on the side of the headache.

Stress or relaxation, hot or cold temperatures, glare, sexual activity, and certain foods may trigger a cluster headache. Cluster sufferers are often smokers, and alcohol is another common trigger. Drinking any kind of alcohol will usually bring on an attack within a few minutes in a patient who is in a cluster-headache cycle, but it will not induce an attack when the patient is in remission.

Cluster headaches affect less than 1 percent of the population and affect men eight to ten times more frequently than they do women. They typically strike men between the ages of 20 and 50 years.

Victor Sanchez, 60, is a heavy smoker. He knows that his smoking may exacerbate his cluster headaches. Though the intense pain nearly paralyzes him several times a year, he continues to smoke. Cigarettes are a longtime addiction he can't shake.

As a small child in Mexico, Victor remembers, he had bad headaches. His parents assumed they stemmed from something he ate because the pain was so severe that he often threw up. He would cry for hours before eventually falling asleep. The next day the pain would be gone. He never knew when it might return.

"In those days, headaches were just headaches," he says. "They had no special names like cluster or migraine. We called them 'jaqueca' [bad headache]."

Sometimes home remedies worked wonders. Taking the advice of villagers, he would suck on a lime hoping to ease the pain. One woman, a fellow headache sufferer, told him to dab a menthol rub on his temple where the pain was most severe. That gave him some relief. He uses it still. It's part of the artillery he turns to when he feels an episode developing.

For many years, Victor coped with the severe pain without help. "I had to learn to function through it," he says. In his mid-50s, he arrived at the headache center at Cleveland Clinic for help. After trying a number of therapies, he now takes verapamil, a calcium-channel blocker used to limit the length of the cluster period and decrease the severity of the attacks. He takes Fiorinol for pain.

When Victor feels his headaches coming on, he "mans the battle stations" – gathering medications, menthol salve, ice bags, and nasal spray – to settle in for a trip to hell, he says. He'll try anything to help him through the pain. "I scramble as soon as I feel it coming. If I can halve the pain, I can deal with it," he says.

Restless and pacing through the house in the grip of an attack, he feels angry and desperate. The right side of his temple pounds, his right sinus fills up, and his right eye weeps. His wife feels helpless, squeezing his hand, massaging his neck. "If it gives me five seconds *of relief, I am grateful," says Victor. He frequently lies on the floor, a handkerchief tied tightly around his head, crying. "It just breaks you," he says. When the episode is over, every muscle in his body aches. "It's exhausting. I feel so helpless."*

Victor is sometimes reluctant to say he has "a headache" because most people don't understand the severity of what he feels.

Treatment

While migraine sufferers tend to retreat to a quiet, dark room, cluster-headache sufferers are usually restless and agitated, and tend to pace or rock back and forth. Because the onset of cluster-headache attacks is rapid and may occur several times a day, the best approach to treatment is with daily preventive drugs. Effective preventive therapy will shorten the length of the cluster period and reduce the number and severity of the daily attacks of pain. Doctors often have to try several medications before the right one is found.

Effective preventive medications include verapamil HCl, prednisone, lithium carbonate, methysergide, and the anti-epileptic drugs divalproex (Depakote) and topiramate (Topamax). High doses of verapamil (480 mg to 720 mg/day) may be necessary. Prednisone and methysergide work quickly and are often used along with verapamil, lithium, or an antiepileptic drug at the onset of the cluster for a quick response, and then tapered while the verapamil, lithium, or antiepileptic drug is continued. Prednisone is usually prescribed at 60 mg/day initially, and then tapered over two to three weeks.

For treatment of the acute cluster attack, the use of 100 percent oxygen by mask at a flow rate of 8 to 10 L/min for up to ten minutes will abort an acute cluster headache in 50 to 60 percent of patients. Ergotamine tartrate, DHE, and any of the triptans usually are very effective in the acute attack but are inappropriate for patients who are suffering several attacks a day. Fortunately, cluster-headache patients do not appear to develop rebound headaches from frequent use of ergotamine tartrate or the triptans, as do migraine sufferers.

Because the attacks come on so quickly, oral agents are not very effective for relief of the pain. Dihydroergotamine (DHE) is often very effective and is used to break an attack. It can be given intravenously in the emergency room or patients can administer it as a nasal spray or by self-injection. While using 100 percent oxygen therapy for ten minutes can often abort a cluster attack, it does not prevent further attacks.

Methysergide (Sansert) is the only drug approved by the U.S. FDA for the treatment of cluster headache, but it is no longer marketed in the United States. (It is still marketed in Canada and Europe.)

Over the years, various surgical procedures have been used to cut branches of the trigeminal nerve or treat the nerve with glycerol, radiation, or radio-frequency waves, but none of these techniques has been very successful. There is hope that new procedures such as deep brain stimulation in the area of the hypothalamus and occipital nerve stimulation may help control these painful headaches, but these are still experimental and need to be studied further. (Occipital nerve stimulation is also being tried in chronic migraine.)

Over the years, both David and Victor have tried numerous medications, hypnotism, acupuncture, and high-flow oxygen therapy – anything that might work.

When the pain begins, both men begin to panic, reaching for medicines or the oxygen mask next to the bed. "I feel totally helpless," says David. "I can't even put my head on the pillow. I just prop myself up and pray."

His wife brings cold compresses and holds his hand, kneeling by his bed. The worst attacks last about two hours. "The beginning is the most desperate time because I know what the whole process is going to be," he says. "I just have to ride it out."

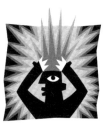

Chapter 5

Headaches in Children and the Elderly, and Other Headaches

Headaches in children

Today's kids are on the go, racing from school to sports practice, sports practice to dance class, dance class to play rehearsal, and then home to study for the next day's exams. All day, every day, is a rush to the finish. Add to that peer pressure, substance abuse, and the high rate of separation and divorce among parents, and it's clear that young people are under more stress than ever before. School is probably the biggest stressor for kids. And yes, straight-A, overachieving students tend to be more at risk for developing headaches than average students.

More than a hundred years ago, British pediatrician William Henry Day developed a theory about why kids have headaches.

One of the first recorded references to headaches in children came in his book *Essays on Disease in Children*, published in 1873. In a chapter devoted entirely to headaches, he stated that nonorganic, nonvascular headaches were the most common type found in children: "Headaches in the young are for the most part due to bad arrangements in their lives." Clearly, though they may be different types of arrangements, "bad arrangements" are still a big problem today.

At Cleveland Clinic, it has been found that headaches occur least frequently in children age 7 and under. For those in this age group who do have head pain, the most common cause is migraine. As children age, the frequency of migraine decreases while the incidence of both tension-type and mixed (tension-type and migraine) headache increases.

By the time they're teens, at least half of all kids have had a headache. Fifteen percent of children and teenagers have tension-type headaches; 5 percent have migraines. Cluster headaches are a rarity in children.

Many will outgrow their headaches when they reach their teens. Boys who have migraines at a young age tend to outgrow them as they enter adolescence, but migraine frequency increases for girls as their hormones change during adolescence.

Children with migraine usually have a family history of migraine. When both parents have a history of migraine, there is a 75 percent chance that the child will also develop migraine.

If only one parent has a history of migraine, the risk drops to 50 percent. Luckily, fewer than 5 percent of those headaches are the result of serious disease or organic problems such as brain tumor, infection, or injury.

Though stress, anxiety, and depression can cause tension-type headaches in children, physical conditions such as eyestrain, poor posture, hunger (skipping breakfast or lunch), and inflammation from diseases of the ears, nose, teeth, neck, jaw, sinuses, or eyes can also cause headaches.

Any child experiencing headache with neurological symptoms such as seizures, loss of consciousness, problems with vision or balance, stiff neck, or fever should receive immediate medical attention. Once serious neurological causes have been eliminated, both the doctors and family can begin to take steps to help control the child's headaches.

Parents must make an effort to discover the cause of their child's pain. Keeping a headache diary can be a great help to your health professional. Help your child record important information like the time of day the headache begins, foods eaten prior to the headache, and specific symptoms. Chatting with the health professionals and teachers at your child's school may give you additional information about possible problems at school.

Headache history remains the primary tool in determining treatment for your child. Take your child to a family physician for a complete physical exam and headache evaluation. This may include a CT scan and MRI. Once a correct headache diagnosis is made, an effective treatment plan can begin. If the headaches become worse or don't respond to treatment, ask your physician for a referral to a pediatric neurologist or headache specialist.

Counseling is an excellent way to help kids learn how to manage stress – an important and necessary life skill. Learning how to prioritize activities, how to exercise and relax (children and teens often respond better than adults do to biofeedback), and how to eat healthfully can go a long way toward helping control headache pain.

Types of pediatric headaches

Primary headaches are those that are not the result of another medical condition. They include:

- Acute, recurrent headaches or migraine. A migraine can be a moderate-to-severe headache that lasts from one to twenty-four hours and occurs two to four times per month. Decreased appetite, dizziness, paleness, blurred vision, upset stomach, nausea, and vomiting are common symptoms. Sensitivity to light, noise, and odors is also common. A small number of pediatric migraine sufferers have abdominal migraines about once a month that include recurrent pain and vomiting.

- **Chronic nonprogressive headaches or tension-type headaches.** These frequent headaches that come and go without causing neurological symptoms are the most common type of headaches in adolescents and are often related to increased stress or an emotional problem.
- **Mixed-headache syndrome.** A combination of migraine and tension-type headaches.

Secondary headaches are the result of another, underlying medical condition. They include:

- **Acute headaches.** Illness, the common cold, fever sinusitis, sore throat, and ear infection are familiar causes of these headaches in children.
- **Chronic progressive headaches.** Headaches that get worse and happen more frequently may be the sign of a disease process in the brain such as hydrocephalus, meningitis, encephalitis, hemorrhage, tumor, blood clots, head trauma, and abscess. These are the least common type of headache and account for less than 2 percent of all children's headaches.

Smaller doses of some of the same medications used to treat headaches in adults are often used to treat children. However, aspirin *should not* be used to treat headaches in children under the age of 15, due to the risk of Reye's syndrome, a rare disorder that children get when they're recovering from such childhood infections as the flu or chicken pox.

Abdominal migraine

This type of migraine, also known as "periodic syndrome," is characterized by recurring attacks of abdominal pain, vomiting, and occasionally vertigo that can last up to seventy-two hours. There is usually a strong family history of migraine in children with this condition, and the typical migraine-preventive medications and antinausea drugs are often helpful in controlling these attacks. This condition should be diagnosed only after abdominal disease has been excluded by various tests.

Headaches in the older population

In the field of headache, the term "elderly" is often applied to persons over the age of 50.

The primary headache conditions – migraine, tension-type, and cluster – almost always begin before age 45. Some headache syndromes are more common in older persons, and a few occur almost exclusively in persons over 50, where common headaches are often associated with other medical conditions. Also, elderly persons are often taking a number of medications, some of which may cause headaches.

When a headache occurs for the first time in someone over the age of 50 or a headache pattern changes in one who has previously suffered with headaches, a complete evaluation is needed to search for an underlying cause.

Migraine, tension-type, and cluster headaches

It is quite rare for **migraine** to occur for the first time in someone over the age of 40. If this happens, the patient must be evaluated for "symptomatic migraine," a migraine-type headache that is due to another underlying condition.

As the migraine sufferer gets older, the attacks tend to become less frequent and less severe. The nausea and general disability associated with migraine usually will lessen as one grows older. Many women whose migraines have had a hormonal trigger will have very few attacks after menopause.

However, migraine variants such as migraine aura without headache, amnesia, and transient migrainous accompaniments (consisting of symptoms such as numbness or tingling in the limbs, blurred vision, clumsiness, or ringing in the ears) occur more commonly in older migraineurs. The visual symptoms tend to last fifteen to sixty minutes and slowly evolve and spread across the field of vision, and then clear. The symptoms are "positive" – being bright and shimmering – and may take on various designs.

The visual defects occurring as a result of lack of blood flow due to hardening of arteries are called transient ischemic attacks. They are usually dark and don't move or spread across the field of vision as do visual symptoms of migraine. They also tend to be shorter in duration than migraine auras, lasting two to five minutes, and usually occur on just one side of the face, a result of disease in the carotid artery system, which supplies blood to the brain.

Other transient migrainous accompaniments are episodes of numbness and tingling in the limbs that slowly spread up or down the extremities. This tingling tends to last twenty to thirty minutes, as does a typical migraine aura. In migraine, the tingling will clear in reverse order, with the area that was involved first clearing last. Symptoms due to lack of blood flow will hit more suddenly, last only five to ten minutes, and will clear in the same order they developed.

When amnesia occurs, it lasts from one to three hours. Sufferers function and act normally but have no recollection for that period of time.

Migraine medications that have vasoconstrictive properties (causing blood vessels to narrow), such as the widely used triptans and ergotamines, must be used with caution in older persons and *should not* be used if there is uncontrolled hypertension or evidence of cerebral, coronary, and peripheral vascular disease. If there is no evidence of significant vascular disease, the triptans are felt to be safe for treating migraine and cluster headaches because they have not been associated with an increased risk of stroke or heart attacks.

Aura symptoms occurring without headache usually do not occur very frequently. Therefore, once the diagnosis is made, daily preventive medication may not be indicated. If it is necessary, the usual preventive drugs used in treating migraine may be effective in the elderly at lower doses. Long-term use of NSAIDs needs to be closely monitored in older persons because such use may lead to kidney damage, worsening of hypertension, and aggravation of underlying cerebral and heart disease.

Tension-type headache may be more prevalent in the elderly and can be attributed to many causes. As in younger persons with tension-type headache, stress and depression are the most common factors behind this condition.

In older individuals, excessive muscle tension in the neck, scalp, and facial muscles may be caused or aggravated by cervical arthritis, poor posture, visual abnormalities, and temporal mandibular joint (the joint between the head and the jaw) disorders. Excessive spasm in those muscles used for chewing may be due to arthritis in the joint, clenching of the teeth, or an abnormal bite because of missing teeth or poorly fitting dentures.

Degenerative arthritis in the cervical spine, which is very common in persons over 50, rarely causes headache unless there is irritation of the nerves in the upper neck. But when someone experiences tenderness over one side of the back of the head, it suggests that the roots of the occipital nerve in the neck may be irritated from disease. If this is the case, an occipital nerve block should give relief.

Degenerative changes at any level of the cervical spine (the neck), however, may be a source of irritation and cause spasms in the neck muscles. An exam will reveal limited range of motion of the neck and tender neck muscles. Poor posture with slouching, rounded shoulders and a forward-positioned head are common in older individuals and may be the cause of pain due to strain, spasm, and tightness in the neck muscles.

Physical therapy aimed at improving range of motion, posture, and balance may be quite helpful for some persons with neck and head pain, and may lessen the need for medications. If stress is an important factor, relaxation techniques, biofeedback, and stress-management skills may be helpful. Preventive medications for tension-type headache such as the tricyclic antidepressants, muscle relaxants, and NSAIDs should be used with caution in the elderly, due to the possibility of excessive sedation and other possible side effects.

Many older persons may experience a **rebound headache** resulting from the frequent use of analgesics. Rebound or "analgesic-maintained headache" can occur with daily or near-daily use of analgesics. Physicians believe that pain medications suppress the brain's own pain-fighting substances – such as endorphins – and sensitize the nerve cells of the brain so that head pain recurs when the patient stops taking the pain medicine. And if the sufferer does not continue taking the medications on a regular basis, the headache comes back: a true vicious cycle. A diagnosis of rebound headache should be considered in patients who awaken every morning with a headache. If they sleep several hours and therefore do not take the offending pain medicine for a while, they will awaken in a withdrawal state.

Cluster headache, like migraine, generally tends to be less of a problem as one ages. Most older persons can safely use the usual preventive medications such as verapamil, lithium, and the antiepileptic drugs. However, prolonged use of prednisone, which is usually very effective in treating cluster headache, can accelerate osteoporosis, elevate blood sugars, and cause easy bruising and gastric complications. As in the case of migraine, drugs with vasoconstrictive properties need to be used with caution. Breathing 100 percent oxygen through a mask may be quite effective in aborting cluster attacks.

Hypnic headache, though very uncommon, occurs mostly in older persons. This type of pain arises at night, awakening the sufferer at about the same time every night with a steady discomfort in the frontal area of the head. The pain of hypnic headache is not as intense as cluster, and the tearing and nasal congestion that commonly accompany cluster headache are absent. Hypnic headaches last one to two hours. Their cause is unknown. After a few months, their frequency may ease. Lithium carbonate, one of the tricyclic antidepressants, or an antiepileptic drug taken at bedtime will usually prevent the attacks.

Temporal (giant-cell) arteritis

Occurring almost exclusively in people over age 50, temporal arteritis (also known as giant-cell arteritis) is a headache caused by inflamed arteries in the head or neck. Although the pain is usually centered in the temples, it can strike any area of the head. The pain is typically a steady ache or a dull, throbbing discomfort.

Temporal arteritis is one of the few headache emergencies, since permanent loss of vision occurs in 20 to 30 percent of those not treated. In addition to the headache, patients often experience fatigue, tiredness, and low-grade fever. They may have stiff and painful muscles in the shoulder and pelvic regions, especially in the morning. Scalp tenderness is also common, and pain with chewing may be experienced.

Temporal arteritis results in an inflammation of medium-sized arteries. Vision loss occurs due to lack of blood flow to the retina and/or the optic nerve, which is caused by narrowing of the artery from the inflammation in the wall of the vessel.

If a patient is experiencing this condition, the sedimentation-rate blood test, which measures inflammation in the body, will be elevated. In addition, a mild anemia is frequently present. To avoid possible vision loss, patients who are suspected of having temporal arteritis should be given prednisone (cortisone) immediately. The headache due to this condition responds quickly and dramatically to high doses of prednisone. A temporal-artery biopsy should also be done to confirm the diagnosis; if the biopsy is negative, prednisone should be discontinued.

Treatment with steroids should be continued for several months and sometimes for a year or more until the temporal arteritis clears up. In addition, the patient needs to be followed clinically and with lab tests while the prednisone dose is gradually decreased over several months. Long-term use of corticosteroids in elderly patients is likely to cause gastric complications, high blood sugars, and osteoporosis, all of which need to be monitored and treated. Calcium supplements, vitamin D, and other therapy to lessen osteoporosis may be necessary. Visual loss and other complications of this disease are very uncommon after four to six weeks of high doses of corticosteroids but can occasionally occur.

Polymyalgia rheumatica (pain and stiffness in shoulder, neck, upper arm, and pelvic muscles) may be associated with temporal arteritis but can occur in its absence. The stiffness and pain is worse during the night and upon awaking. Headache is usually not a prominent feature. Polymyalgia rheumatica will respond quickly to *low doses* of prednisone in the range of 5 to 20 mg daily.

Subdural hematoma

Subdural hematomas (bleeding between the skull and the brain) occur more frequently in older persons. Bleeding may develop after a minor head injury, when the head is jolted, or even after vigorous sneezing or coughing. Persons taking daily aspirin or other blood-thinners are also more prone to develop bleeding from a minimal head injury. The bleeding is usually caused by a rupture of a vein and may take several days or weeks for symptoms to develop after the injury.

Headache resulting from subdural hematoma is usually a dull, mild discomfort in the head. Other symptoms include drowsiness, confusion, and personality changes. Small subdural hematomas can be observed, and these bruises will usually heal by themselves without the need for surgery. But a large hematoma, coupled with the presence of confusion and drowsiness, means that surgery is needed.

Trigeminal neuralgia

Ninety percent of the cases of trigeminal neuralgia (sharp pains in the forehead, face, or jaw) occur in persons over 40 years of age. Also called tic douloureux, this condition is due to irritation of the trigeminal nerve (fifth cranial nerve). When it occurs in a younger person, it is usually due to a neurological disease, often multiple sclerosis, and less often an infection or tumor.

The trigeminal nerve has three branches. Usually the second and third branches, which supply sensation to the cheek and jaw, are affected. The sharp, jabbing pains occur for a few seconds at a time in a repetitive, wavelike crescendo pattern. Pain is induced or triggered by touching or stimulation of the face, such as when shaving, chewing, laughing, or brushing teeth. Because of the facial area affected, this condition is sometimes confused with cluster headache, but cluster pain is not triggered by touching the face and is a steady pain, with each attack lasting thirty minutes to two hours.

The cause of trigeminal neuralgia may be due to compression of the root of the nerve by an artery in the posterior part of the brain, or it can be caused by any irritation along the main nerve or any of the three branches. Previous viral infection involving the nerve may also be a culprit.

Medications will usually control this condition. Anticonvulsant drugs such as carbamazepine (Tegretol), gabapentin (Neurontin), or pregabalin (Lyrica) are usually effective. But if medication doesn't control the pain, surgical approaches need to be considered.

Herpes zoster and post-herpetic neuralgia

Herpes zoster (shingles) is due to the reactivation of the dormant varicella (chicken pox) virus in nerve cells. When it involves the trigeminal nerve tissue, the face is affected – specifically the eye, where the pain is severe and visual loss may occur. In addition, blisterlike lesions may appear after several days. Altered immunity due to chronic illness or the use of corticosteroids or other immunosuppressive drugs may be a factor in reactivation of the dormant virus. Early treatment with antiviral agents such as acyclovir (Zovirax), famciclovir (Famvir), or valacyclovir (Valtrex) may help control the pain and eruption, and prevent eye involvement.

Post-herpetic neuralgia is pain that persists for more than three months after the skin lesions have healed. It tends to be more common in older persons and may occur in up to 50 percent of those afflicted in their 60s and 70s. Antidepressants and the antiepileptic drugs have been helpful in controlling post-herpetic neuralgia pain.

Other medical conditions associated with headache

Hypertensive headache may occur if the diastolic (lower) blood pressure is consistently over 120 mm of mercury. This headache is typically a generalized throbbing pain that is worse in the early morning hours or upon waking, and tends to ease as one gets up and moves about. Migraine headache however is frequently exacerbated by mildly elevated levels of blood pressure. Diastolic levels in the range of 90 to 110 may aggravate the underlying migraine pattern.

Sleep apnea, which may cause low blood oxygen and/or retention of carbon dioxide, can cause headache upon waking and will generally ease as one gets up and moves about. Endocrine abnormalities such as hypothyroidism (underactive thyroid), hyperthyroidism (overactive thyroid), and hypercalcemia (high blood-calcium level) can also cause headaches. Hypoglycemia (low blood sugar) can cause headache, but is usually associated with other symptoms such as sweating, palpitations, and hunger.

Malignancies – primary brain tumors and metastatic brain lesions – are more prevalent in older persons and need to be considered in anyone experiencing the onset of a new headache. The headache associated with brain tumors is usually not severe. If the brain lesion is large, obstructing the flow of cerebral-spinal fluid, the pain will be worse when the patient sits or stands upright.

Connective-tissue diseases, anemia, high blood count, high blood-platelet count, and electrolyte abnormalities are other conditions that may be associated with headache or can worsen a preexisting headache. Acute glaucoma may be associated with a severe pain in and around the eye that comes on rather abruptly and is accompanied by visual blurring and eye redness.

Medications that may cause headache

Elderly persons tend to take more medicines; therefore, it is very important to thoroughly review all the medications ingested. This is especially true if the headache is of recent onset or the headache pattern has changed and there has been a recent change in medicines.

Commonly used medications that may cause headache include any of the vasodilating drugs that are used for heart disease or hypertension. The most common offending drugs include nitroglycerin, isosorbide (Isordil), nifedipine (Procardia), hydralazine (Apresoline), and prazosin (Minipress). Nonsteroidal drugs, particularly indomethacin (Indocin) and diclofenac (Voltaren), can cause headache. Some other drugs that may produce headaches include the estrogens, H2 blockers such as Tagamet, various sulfa preparations, tetracyclines, cyclosporine, tamoxifen, and danazol.

Anyone over age 50 who develops a new kind of headache or experiences a change in headache pattern needs to be investigated for an underlying condition that may be the cause or an exacerbating factor. Several headache syndromes occur almost exclusively in older persons, and medications may be the cause. Many medications taken by younger headache patients need to be used with caution because of other complicating medical conditions that might be present.

Other headaches

There are more than 150 different types of headaches that have been described. Let's take a look at some of the most common.

Allergy headaches are caused by seasonal allergens like pollen or mold. Allergies to food are not usually a factor. Nasal congestion and watery eyes usually accompany this headache. The use of antihistamine medication or cortisone-related topical nasal sprays might help. Desensitization injections may also provide relief.

Arthritis headaches are caused by inflammation in the temporal mandibular (jaw) joint or in the bony structures of the neck. Use of muscle relaxants and anti-inflammatory drugs will help this condition.

Caffeine-withdrawal headaches are caused by dilation of the blood vessels that occurs for several days after consumption of large quantities of caffeine. Stopping or cutting down caffeine consumption may be needed.

Exertional headaches are triggered by physical activities such as running, weightlifting, and sexual intercourse, and typically affect otherwise healthy people who have not previously been prone to headaches. Interestingly, exercise is something that makes an existing migraine worse while tension-type headache tends to improve with exercise. These headaches generally affect younger people, come on quickly, and can be very severe.

Bilateral and throbbing, they can last from a few minutes up to twenty-four hours and tend to stop when the activity is over. The exact causes are unknown but could involve dilated blood vessels, overly contracted muscles, and the release of pain-producing substances. Patients who are involved in intense athletic competitions and are already on a preventive headache drug may have to check with their doctor regarding the possibility of increasing the medication prior to a competition. Anti-inflammatory drugs work best for most people. On rare occasions, exertional headaches could be caused by organic disease and should be checked out by a physician.

Hangover headaches are caused by excessive alcohol consumption. Alcohol causes blood vessels to swell or dilate, but metabolic products resulting from alcohol use also contribute to the headache pain and sweating the morning after. Because alcohol acts as a diuretic, it leads to dehydration. Before imbibing, eat some honey – it's rich in vitamin B_6 and can reduce hangover symptoms. Other tricks include staying away from red wine and alternating nonalcoholic beverages with alcoholic beverages. Tomato juice or any fruit juice high in fructose allows the body to burn alcohol faster. As the evening progresses, keep the fluids flowing, take ibuprofen, or drink a cup of coffee: Caffeine eases dilated blood vessels.

Hunger headaches are caused by low blood sugar. This causes dilation of the blood vessels. Oversleeping, dieting, and skipping meals are the main triggers. Eating balanced meals on a regular timetable will prevent these headaches.

Sex headache is caused by sexual activity. Paradoxically, other headache sufferers find that sexual activity can relieve their headaches. There are two types of this "orgasmic headache." In the first type, excitement during intercourse causes muscle contraction in the neck and head that may lead to head pain. The second type is a vascular headache – a very severe headache, usually behind the eyes, just prior to orgasm. This may be a response to an increase in blood pressure during which the blood vessels dilate. This benign headache occurs most often in men. Sometimes, migraine sufferers may need to take migraine medications such as triptans before intercourse. This type of headache during intercourse may be a symptom of a more serious problem and should be thoroughly investigated.

Sinus headache is believed to be a rare condition. Many people who think they have a sinus headache may actually be dealing with a migraine. True sinusitis symptoms include post-nasal drainage, congestion, and facial pressure with taste and smell being affected. When sinus disease is the cause of the headache, fever is usually present. Sinus disease rarely causes chronic, recurring headaches.

Temporomandibular joint (TMJ) headache is one of the many symptoms of temporomandibular disease, which can be caused by injuries to the jaw, malocclusion (poor bite), the presence of osteoarthritis or rheumatoid arthritis, stress, and jaw-clenching. Women between the ages of 20 and 40 are the most common sufferers.

The temporomandibular joint is the hinge joint that connects the lower jaw to the temporal bone of the skull in front of both ears. This flexible joint allows the jaw to move from side to side and up and down as necessary for chewing, yawning, and speech. The muscles attached to and around the jaw joint control the position and movement of the jaw. Jaw and headache pain occur when the joint area becomes worn out or moves out of place.

Symptoms include:

- Facial pain
- Decreased range of motion
- Clicking and popping in the jaw joint
- Tooth pain
- Ear pain
- Tinnitus
- Stuffiness
- Headache

Sometimes it's difficult to diagnose temporomandibular disease because other conditions such as toothache, sinusitis, arthritis, or gum disease can cause similar symptoms. The first step is a visit to the dentist, where a panoramic x-ray of the jaw allows a dentist to view the entire jaw, joint, and teeth. A magnetic resonance imaging test (MRI) or a computer tomography (CT) test can also be helpful. The MRI reveals whether the soft tissue is in the proper position when the jaw moves. A CT scan reveals the bony detail of the joint.

Treatment involves NSAIDs like ibuprofen (Advil, Motrin), naproxen sodium (Aleve), or aspirin to relieve headache and muscle pain. Muscle relaxants, anti-anxiety drugs, and antidepressants may help. The most effective approach is to wear a specially made "bite guard" at night to take pressure off the joint.

Fibromyalgia

Nine years ago, special-needs teacher Kathy Dowling began to ache all over. In addition, excruciating headaches made her crawl into a quiet, dark location in the school's infirmary, looking for relief. Light and sound were big elements. Some days, with twenty-five children in her classroom, she'd have to call for a colleague to take over while she went into a dark room to lie down and put something over her eyes.

She hopped from doctor to doctor, specialist to specialist. "It was brand new at that point," says Kathy of the pain she experienced.

"No one knew what to do with it." Very little information existed. She said it was tough on family relationships as well – sympathy was at a minimum. "I looked perfectly normal, but I was exhausted and aching. I could sleep all day. Xanax was a miracle drug for me."

Six million Americans have been diagnosed with fibromyalgia, a condition characterized by painful aching in the muscles, tendons, and joints all over the body. In addition to widespread pain and fatigue, many patients report chronic tension-type and migraine headaches.

Fibromyalgia is a "functional" illness, which means that the symptoms are real, not imagined. Yet medical tests turn out normal for patients suffering from this disease, which makes diagnosing it frustrating for both doctor and patient. Another difficulty in diagnosing this condition is that the symptoms mimic those of lupus and chronic fatigue syndrome. Symptoms tend to arise during times of stress, depression, anxiety, lack of sleep, lack of exercise, and traumatic life experiences. Also, symptoms seem to flare during damp, cold weather. During flare-ups, the pain is relentless; during remission, it is less intense.

Fibromyalgia affects more women than men. Typically people first develop symptoms in their 20s or 30s. Though it is not progressive, crippling, or life-threatening, without proper care, fibromyalgia can cause complete exhaustion and despair.

There is no cure, but fibromyalgia can be managed. Unfortunately, the disease is not well understood and many physicians do not understand how prevalent it is. Many patients see an average of three doctors and may undergo unnecessary testing before a diagnosis is made.

In nearly all cases, the patient is enduring considerable stress or an overwhelmingly busy lifestyle at the onset of fibromylagia. Stress contributes to disturbed sleep patterns, and without enough sleep the body doesn't produce the chemicals necessary to control or regulate pain. A lack of these pain-regulating chemicals results in tenderness in the upper back and forearms, leading to the symptoms of fibromyalgia.

Physical or emotional illness can also contribute to the onset of the disease; an infection may cause changes in body chemistry that lead to pain and sleeplessness as well as worry and anxiety. And some researchers believe that fibromyalgia is related to extremely sensitive nerve cells and that neurotransmitters (chemicals in the brain) may be out of whack.

The American College of Rheumatology lists the following criteria for a fibromyalgia diagnosis:

1. **Widespread pain for at least three months** in the following spots: the left and right sides of the body, above the waist, below the waist, and axial pain—pain in the cervical spine (thoracic pain) or in the low back or anterior chest wall.

2. **The presence of eleven tender points** among eighteen specified sites on the back of the head, upper back and neck, upper chest, elbows, hips, and knees. People who have fibromyalgia have abnormal sensitivity when light pressure is applied to these areas of the body.

Many other conditions such as irritable bowel syndrome, dizziness, and temporomandibular joint dysfunction may also be present, making diagnosis and treatment even more difficult. Both tension-type and migraine headaches are common.

Studies have shown that aerobic exercise can have a positive impact on fibromyalgia sufferers. Cardiovascular fitness training, electromyogram biofeedback, hypnotherapy, electroacupuncture, and cognitive-behavioral therapy have also been shown to be helpful. In addition, because so many sufferers also experience depression, cognitive-behavioral therapy empowers patients to care for themselves through counseling and classes.

Medications such as antidepressants and muscle relaxants can relieve sleep and pain symptoms. Over-the-counter acetaminophen (Tylenol) can ease headache and muscular pain. NSAIDs – aspirin, ibuprofen (Advil, Motrin), and naproxen sodium (Aleve, Anaprox) – and tricyclic antidepressants used in tandem with other medications such as pregabalin (Lyrica)

– which was recently approved by the FDA for the treatment of fibromyalgia – may be helpful. But drugs alone do not seem to manage the pain of fibromyalgia.

As with all illnesses, products claiming total fatigue relief abound. Beware of snake-oil salesmen preying on the desperate.

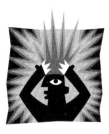

Chapter 6

Alternatives

Integrative medicine merges complementary and alternative forms of medicine with traditional medicine to help prevent disease, decrease suffering, and empower patients to take better care of themselves. This new way of looking at health care is becoming more and more accepted in medical communities across America.

The Center for Integrative Medicine at Cleveland Clinic helps patients learn to control headache pain by trying a variety of nonpharmaceutical and behavioral therapies such as relaxation techniques and lifestyle changes.

Acupuncture and acupressure

These two forms of therapy originated in China more than 3,000 years ago. Why acupuncture works is still unknown, but it is believed that the insertion of fine needles into points along meridians that run through the body is an attempt to release "chi," the body's life-energy force. This stimulation may release certain endorphins when acupuncture points are stimulated.

Though physicians have not embraced acupuncture because of the lack of documented scientific validity, several small studies have shown that acupuncture has reduced the need for headache medications as well reducing headache frequency. The therapy is not harmful.

Acupressure is similar to acupuncture, but instead of using needles, a type of finger-pressure massage is used to stimulate pressure points on the body. This is also thought to release blocked energy flow or "chi."

Biofeedback

Because many scientific studies have shown the positive effects of biofeedback, this type of therapy has become widely accepted in many traditional headache and pain centers around the country. Patients who try this must be willing to make the commitment to the therapy because they will become very involved in their own headache treatment.

There are three forms of biofeedback:

- Thermal or temperature feedback. This helps regulate the blood flow to the hands. For instance, by monitoring a thermometer taped to a finger, a patient learns to use relaxation exercises to make the temperature of the finger rise. Patients learn how to gain control over their physiological reactions in order to use the same relaxation responses during periods of regular daily stress.

- Muscular biofeedback (electromyography). This positions sensors on the skin over the forehead, neck, and shoulder muscles. Using relaxation techniques, patients learn to decrease the tension in these muscles in ways they can apply during normal daily activities.
- Brain-wave biofeedback (electroencephalography). This involves placing sensors on the scalp. Here, patients learn to slow brain activity through a variety of relaxation techniques.

Learning to relax can reduce unwanted emotional responses to stress, an unavoidable part of daily life. Unfortunately, too much stress can interfere with daily relationships and activities, and lead to headaches, anxiety, and depression. With practice, individuals can learn biofeedback methods on their own. Time in a quiet, soothing place should be set aside each day for this purpose.

Breathing

How you breathe is an important part of how you deal with stress, and deep breathing is the key to decreasing tension.

Learning abdominal breathing allows you to take air deep into your lungs by contracting and expanding the diaphragm.

Here's how to do it:

1. Sit down.
2. Place one hand on your abdomen.
3. Breathe in slowly through the nose.
4. Count to seven as you inhale. Try to fill up your lower lungs with air. Your abdomen and chest should rise.
5. Exhale on another count of seven. Slowly push all the air out of your lungs. Your abdomen will fall.
6. Repeat this exercise several times.

When your breathing and heart rate slow down, you will become relaxed. Do you feel calm?

Herbs and vitamins

Herbs do not have magical or mystical properties. Some have been studied and can be considered safe and effective. However, others are not safe and may cause lasting harm or even death. They may also interact with prescription and nonprescription medications. Check with a health-care professional before using any type of dietary supplement or herbal product.

Many herbal headache remedies – including cannabis (marijuana), passionflower, skullcap, hops, ginger, and the bark of the white willow tree – are credited with relieving or reducing headache pain. Feverfew, a member of the chrysan-themum family, is the most popular. Its leaves, dried for use as a tea or in capsule form, contain a chemical that helps the body use serotonin, an important brain chemical, more effectively.

A study by an international research team at Albert Einstein College of Medicine of Yeshiva University has found success in the war on migraines with butterbur, another herb used for medicinal purposes since ancient times. Both butterbur and feverfew work as migraine preventatives, but they may cause stomach upset. Also, locating supplies of these herbal remedies with consistent potencies may be a challenge.

Magnesium has been used intravenously for treatment of acute migraine, and daily oral use at a dose of 400 to 1200 mg has been occasionally helpful in reducing the severity and frequency of migraine. Magnesium oxide at 400 to 800 mg a day is the usual daily dose.

Riboflavin (vitamin B_2) has been reported in one study to have been effective in reducing the frequency of migraine. The dose used was 400 mg.

Massage
Massage helps relieve tension and muscle tightness, and lifts your mood. You can easily learn some massage techniques on your own or get a massage from a licensed professional.

Meditation

This method involves calming your body and mind while focusing on a single word, phrase, or image, or on your own breathing. The practice of meditation can be traced back thousands of years to ancient Buddhist and Hindu practices. These days, its methods are also used to complement modern medical therapies. Studies published in mainstream medical journals show that meditation is an effective stress-reducer.

In one study, patients with chronic pain (including headaches) experienced significant decreases in pain and reduced their reliance on painkiller drugs after a ten-week program of meditation and yoga. Here's how to do it.

Begin by sitting in a chair or on the floor with your legs crossed in front of you. Start out with ten to fifteen minutes of meditation each day, then increase to twenty to thirty minutes daily when you feel comfortable.

Here's how to do it:

1. Close your eyes.
2. Breathe smoothly and evenly. You can slowly count breaths (from one to four, then start again) or repeat a word in your mind as you exhale.
3. Imagine your body at peace. Relax any tense spots.
4. If you get distracted, refocus and continue to meditate.

When you have finished, take some time to stretch or sit quietly. Be patient; meditation takes time to master, but those who are willing to learn and practice these techniques will reap great benefits.

Nutritional counseling

Our daily dietary habits play a huge role in the prevention and treatment of many chronic conditions. A visit with a registered dietitian can help patients learn how to practice preventive nutrition with a "whole foods" approach.

Progressive muscle relaxation

This technique involves the tightening and releasing of different muscles until they're relaxed. As you do this, you learn to recognize which muscles are tense. Take fifteen minutes out of your day to relax yourself from head to toe.

Here's how to do it:

1. Sit or lie down and close your eyes.
2. Start with the feet and calf muscles: Slowly tighten muscles for about five seconds, then relax them for about twenty seconds. Repeat this action five times.
3. Repeat Step 2 for the following muscle groups: thighs and buttocks; abdomen and chest; fingers and arms; shoulders and neck; face and head.

4. Finish by relaxing your whole body. Breathe deeply and slowly. Open your eyes.

Visualization

Use your imagination to transport yourself to a calm, quiet place of comfort. Imagine yourself skipping stones at the beach on a beautiful summer day, watching the sun set over the mountains, or walking through a garden of fragrant roses. Some people enjoy listening to tapes of soothing music or nature sounds.

Visualization can stimulate changes in bodily functions such as heart rate, blood pressure, and respiratory patterns. Research has shown that it may decrease depression, stress, and anxiety; enhance sleep; improve the immune system; and boost self-confidence. It can be done almost anywhere, anytime.

Here's how to do it:

1. Close your eyes.
2. Imagine a calm and relaxing scene or event.
3. Notice all the details, including smells and sounds.
4. Do this until you become relaxed.

Yoga

Yoga is a helpful stretching, breathing, and meditative exercise with numerous physical, mental, emotional, and spiritual benefits. There are many books available on how to practice yoga on your own, and classes in churches and community centers abound.

Does wrinkle-reducer also reduce headaches?

Under the trade name Botox, injections of botulinum toxin type A (BTX-A) have been used cosmetically to remove facial wrinkles, but recent research indicates that it may also have applications in migraine care. BTX-A is a neurotoxin that weakens muscles by blocking the release of acetylcholine, a substance that transmits messages to the muscles. Recent studies have shown that BTX-A also inhibits release of several different chemical substances from the trigeminal nerve endings, and this effect may be the basis of relief in migraine. Some headache sufferers who received Botox injections for wrinkles discovered that they were no longer having headaches. In a clinical trial conducted by Botox manufacturer Allergan, migraine sufferers who underwent Botox injections in the neck and head area reported a significant reduction in attacks. There are several ongoing studies at this time and the overall response rate in migraine seems to be about 50 percent.

However, be aware that Allergan is the *only* company authorized to sell Botox. If you want to try this neurotoxin, make sure you are getting the real thing.

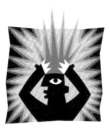

Chapter 7

Headache Questions and Answers*

Q: What causes migraine, and how can I treat it?

A: Generally, migraine begins as a dull ache and then develops into a constant throbbing and pulsating pain that you may feel at the temples as well as at the front or back of one or both sides of the head. The pain is usually accompanied by a combination of nausea, vomiting, and sensitivity to light and noise. Migraine pain and the other symptoms are worsened by physical activity. Some people (about 15 percent of migraine sufferers) experience an aura before an attack. Migraine is an inherited condition and the cause is believed to be due to chemical reactions in the brain. Treatment for migraine may include over-the-counter or prescription medications as well as self-help techniques such as relaxation training and biofeedback.

Q: What is an aura?

A: About 15 percent of people with migraine experience an "aura," which is a manifestation of visual or neurological symptoms that occur before a migraine headache. You may see wavy or jagged lines, dots, or flashing lights, or you might have tunnel vision or blind spots in one or both eyes. The aura can include visual or auditory hallucinations and disruptions in smell (such as strange odors), taste, or touch. Other symptoms include numbness, a "pins-and-needles" sensation, or difficulty in recalling or speaking the correct word. These visual and neurological events may last as long as sixty minutes but will fade as the headache begins.

Q: What is a trigger?

A: Certain physical or environmental factors, such as foods, hormonal changes, weather, and stress, can lead to or "trigger" a migraine in a susceptible person. However, it's important to remember that triggers are different for everyone. That's why, to help prevent migraine attacks, you need to figure out which triggers affect you and which ones don't. Keeping a headache diary is an effective way to track triggers, and it will help you talk to your health-care professional about your condition.

Q: Does weather affect migraines?

A: Bright sunshine, conditions of heat and humidity, and drastic changes in barometric pressure may "trigger" a migraine attack in some migraineurs. However, studies have shown that weather is not always a trigger for everyone who has migraines.

Q: Is there an increased risk of stroke for migraine sufferers?

A: While the severity of a migraine attack often causes patients to fear they are having a stroke, the likelihood of a migraine causing a stroke is very slim. That is not to say that migraine sufferers cannot have a stroke associated with their migraines. In persons under age 40, the most common associated factor for stroke is migraine headache. However, over the course of a person's normal life span, the occurrence of migraine headache may actually be associated with a reduced risk of dying from heart disease.

Q: What is the link between migraine and hormones?

A: Hormones initiate and regulate many of your body's functions, keeping your body in balance within a constantly changing environment. In women, when the levels of female hormones in the body are unbalanced – during menstruation, pregnancy, or menopause – the imbalance can lead to more migraine attacks. In fact, about three-quarters of all women with migraine report that their attacks are related to the menstrual cycle. There is also recent evidence that estrogens have an effect on the functioning of nerve cells in the brain.

Q: What are acute medications for migraine?

A: Acute medications – sometimes referred to as acute abortive medications – are used to treat the pain of the headache after it has started. Examples of acute abortive medications include over-the-counter medications, NSAIDs (nonsteroidal anti-inflammatory drugs), ergots, and triptans.

Q: What are the triptans?

A: Triptans are the newest class of abortive medications targeted to treat migraine. In addition to being vasoconstrictors (which narrow the arteries), they moderate some chemical reactions in the brain. Triptans work on receptors in your brain, helping to restore the balance of a neurotransmitter called serotonin. Changing levels of serotonin are thought to be a main cause of a migraine attack.

Q: Are over-the-counter medications for migraine effective?

A: Over-the-counter (OTC) medications may be effective in relieving mild to moderate pain and associated symptoms of migraine. However, you should see your doctor before beginning any treatment regimen for migraine. These medications should not be used more than twice a week.

Q: What are preventive medications for migraine?

A: Preventive medications for migraine – often referred to as "prophylactic" treatments – are taken on a daily basis and are used to reduce the frequency, severity, and length of migraine attacks. Most preventive migraine medications were initially developed to treat other diseases, such as seizures, depression, or hypertension. Examples of preventive medications include antiepileptic medications, antidepressants, beta-blockers, calcium-channel blockers, and NSAIDs.

Q: Why are anticonvulsants used to treat migraine?

A: Most preventive migraine medications were initially developed to treat diseases like seizures, depression, or hypertension. During the past few years, there has been an increased interest in antiepileptic drugs (sometimes referred to as "anticonvulsants") for the prevention of migraine, as both epilepsy and migraine may be caused by similar reactions starting in the brain cells.

Q: Why are antidepressants used to treat migraine?

A: Antidepressants are typically used to treat people suffering from depression. They may also reduce migraine frequency by regulating the levels of serotonin and other chemicals in the brain.

Q: What alternative therapies are used to treat migraine?

A: The term "alternative therapies" is often used to describe treatments considered outside the scope of conventional Western medicine. Examples of alternative therapy include acupuncture, acupressure, and yoga. Another common alternative treatment is herbal therapy since some herbs are believed to relieve headache pain. Always discuss alternative therapies with your doctor before proceeding with them.

Q: What causes a tension-type headache, and how can I treat it?

A: Tension-type headaches occur randomly and are often the result of temporary stress, anxiety, fatigue, or anger. Symptoms include soreness in your temples, a tightening, bandlike sensation around your head (a "viselike" ache), a pulling feeling, pressure sensations, and contracting head and neck muscles. The headache may begin in your forehead or temples, or the back of your head and neck. The pain of tension-type headache is usually not as severe as migraine and is not accompanied by the other common migraine symptoms. Treatment for tension-type headache may include over-the-counter or prescription medications as well as self-help techniques such as relaxation training and biofeedback.

Q: What causes a cluster headache, and how can I treat it?

A: Cluster headache gets its name because the attacks come in groups. The pain arrives with little, if any, warning and is always on one side of the head. There may be two to three attacks a day for a period of several weeks and then the attacks cease. A tearing or bloodshot eye and a runny nose on the side of the headache may also accompany the pain. Cluster headache, believed to be caused by chemical reactions in the brain, has been described as the most severe and intense of any headache type. Treatment for cluster headache includes prescription medication and oxygen.

Q: What causes a sinus headache, and how can I treat it?

A: When a sinus becomes inflamed, usually as the result of an allergic reaction, an infection, or rarely, a tumor, the inflammation will cause a localized pain. If your headache is truly caused by a sinus blockage, such as an infection, you will probably have a fever. A CT scan or possibly an x-ray will confirm a sinus blockage. Your physician's treatment might include antibiotics for the infection as well as antihistamines or decongestants.

Q: What causes a rebound headache, and how can I treat it?

A: A pattern of taking acute headache medications too often (more than two days per week) or in excessive amounts (more than the label or a doctor advises) can lead to a condition known as rebound headache. With rebound headache, your medications not only stop relieving pain, they actually begin to cause headaches. Doctors treat rebound headache by tapering the medication that is being overused, sometimes by gradually substituting a different type of treatment or medication. Stopping may be a challenge, but regularly overusing a medication increases the potential for serious side effects. Consult a physician if you regularly use headache medications more than two days per week or more than the label advises.

Q: What is biofeedback?

A: Biofeedback is a self-help treatment that uses special equipment to monitor your body's involuntary physical responses such as breathing, pulse, heart rate, temperature, muscle tension, and brain activity. Biofeedback helps you refine and perfect your relaxation exercises by learning to control the physical responses that are related to stress. An important benefit to learning biofeedback is that, once the technique has been mastered, you don't need the equipment anymore.

Q: Are headaches hereditary?

A: According to estimates, approximately 29.5 million people in the United States suffer from migraine. Migraine is an inherited condition; four out of five migraineurs report a family history of migraine. Scientists are not sure whether this is truly genetic or a family predisposition. Despite the uncertainty, studies show that a child has a 50 percent chance of having migraine if one parent suffers from the condition and a 75 percent chance if both parents suffer.

Q: Can children get headaches?

A: Definitely. By the time they reach high school, most young people have experienced some type of headache. However, once your child's physician discovers the cause and type of the headache, many safe and effective approaches or medications can prevent a headache from occurring or stop it after it has attacked.

Q: What type of doctor should I see to diagnose and treat my headache?

A: When seeking treatment for your headache, start with your primary care physician. Discuss your doctor's experience and approach to headaches, including methods of classification, diagnosis, and treatment. Your doctor may recommend you to a headache specialist, depending upon your symptoms or other physical conditions (diabetes, allergies, etc.) that require a more comprehensive and inclusive approach to your headache. Upon request, the National Headache Foundation will provide a list of NHF physician members in your state.

* Material in "Questions and Answers" used with permission of the National Headache Foundation. For more information on headache causes and treatments, visit www.headaches.org.

Appendix

Dispelling Migraine Myths*

Myth: It's all in your head.

Fact: Migraine is a legitimate neurobiological disease with the same validity as such medical disorders as hypertension, diabetes, asthma, and epilepsy.

More than 29.5 million Americans suffer from migraine, with women being affected three times as often than men. It is most commonly experienced between the ages of 15 and 55, and 70 percent to 80 percent of sufferers have a family history of migraine. However, less than half of all migraine sufferers have received a diagnosis of migraine from their health-care providers. Migraine is often misdiagnosed as sinus headache or tension-type headache.

The pain of migraine occurs when excited brain cells trigger the trigeminal nerve to release chemicals that irritate and cause swelling of blood vessels on the surface of the brain. These swollen blood vessels send pain signals to the brainstem, an area of the brain that processes pain information. The pain of migraine is a referred pain, typically felt around the eye or temple area. Pain can also occur in the face, sinus, jaw, or neck area.

Myth: Migraine is just a bad headache.

Fact: Headache is only one symptom of this disease.

Other symptoms include nausea, vomiting, aura (warning symptoms of an attack, such as seeing light spots), sensitivity to light and sound, numbness, and difficulty speaking. A migraine attack can last for hours or days. Attacks can be so debilitating that 150 million days of work are lost each year in the U.S. due to head pain.

Myth: Migraine doesn't run in families.

Fact: Migraines can be hereditary.

If one parent has migraine, a child has a 50 percent chance of also having the disease. If both parents have migraine, there's a 75 percent chance. If even a distant relative has migraine, there's a 20 percent chance the child will develop the disease.

Myth: Migraines are caused by stress.

Fact: Migraine is a biologically based disorder.

It is not caused by stress (or psychological disorders). However, stress is a commonly recognized trigger. Stress can be physical or emotional. It can be good or bad. It is an unavoidable part of modern life.

Migraine sufferers are thought to have highly sensitized brains. In times of emotional stress, certain chemicals are released that provoke the vascular changes that can cause a migraine attack. Factors related to stress included anxiety, worry, shock, depression, excitement, and mental fatigue. After a stressful period there may be a letdown, which can, in itself, trigger a migraine headache.

Myth: Exercise just makes migraine worse.
Fact: For those who suffer from chronic recurring migraines, exercise can either provoke an attack or lessen the frequency and severity of the headaches.

Maintaining a regular exercise program can reduce the number of headache attacks and contribute to overall good health. If exercise or physical strain induces a headache, it's important to see a health-care provider.

Myth: Dietary supplements are not helpful in the treatment of migraine.
Fact: Those suffering from frequent migraines may have low magnesium levels.

Magnesium has a relaxant effect on smooth muscle, such as the smooth muscles in blood vessels. Daily supplementation of 500 to 700 mg increases the body's magnesium level. Riboflavin (vitamin B_2) assists nerve cells in the production of ATP, an energy-producing substance that is essential for many chemical reactions that occur in the body. High doses of riboflavin

(400 mg are recommended) may reverse the "energy crisis" that cells experience during migraine attacks.

Myth: Migraine is unrelated to sleep.
Fact: Migraine can be triggered by lack of sleep.

It's best to go to sleep at the same time every night and wake up the same time each morning, including on weekends. Doing so maintains the body's natural circadian rhythm.

Myth: Migraines cannot be triggered by such stimuli as smoke, smells, or perfume.
Fact: Certain fumes, vapors, odors, and perfumes *can* trigger a migraine headache. Being in public places that are smoke-filled or poorly ventilated can result in a migraine attack.

Myth: Migraineurs should avoid caffeine.
Fact: For certain migraine sufferers, caffeine can trigger an attack. For others, caffeine is a migraine inhibitor.

Keeping a headache diary can help you determine whether caffeine helps or hurts your migraine. Caffeine is an ingredient in coffee, tea, chocolate, colas and certain other soft drinks, and some pain-relieving and acute migraine medications.

* Material in "Dispelling Migraine Myths" used with permission of the National Headache Foundation. For more information on headache causes and treatments, visit www.headaches.org.

References for "Dispelling Migraine Myths"

Seymour Diamond, M.D., *Diagnosing and Managing Headaches*, Professional Communications, Inc., 2004.

Seymour Diamond, M.D., and Mary A. Franklin, *Headache Through the Ages*, Professional Communications, Inc., 2005.

R.B. Lipton, M.D.; H. Göbel, M.D., Ph.D.; K.M. Einhäupl, M.D.; K. Wilks, M.D.; and A. Mauskop, M.D., "Petasites hybridus root (butterbur) is an effective preventive treatment for migraine," *Neurology*; 63:2240-2244, 2004.

J. Schoenen, J. Jacquy, and M. Lenaerts, "Effectiveness of high dose riboflavin in migraine prophylaxis. A randomized controlled trial," *Neurology*; 50:466-470, 1998.

C. David Tollison and Robert S. Kunkel, M.D., *Headache: Diagnosis and Treatment*, Williams & Wilkins, Baltimore 1993.

Resources

Headache Organizations

American Academy of Neurology
1080 Montreal Avenue, St. Paul, Minnesota 55116 / 651-695-1940

American Headache Society
19 Mantua Road, Mount Royal, New Jersey 08061
856-423-0043 / fax: 856-423-0082 / e-mail: ahshq@talley.com

Cleveland Clinic Neurological Institute
Center for Headache and Pain
9500 Euclid Avenue, T33, Cleveland, Ohio 44195 / 216-444-5559
http://cms.clevelandclinic.org/neuroscience

MAGNUM
(Migraine Awareness Group: A National Understanding for Migraineurs)
113 South Saint Asaph Street, Suite 300, Alexandria, Virginia 22314
703-739-9384 / fax: 703-739-2432

National Headache Foundation
820 N. Orleans, Suite 217, Chicago, Illinois 60610-3132
888-NHF-5552 or 773-388-6399 / e-mail: info@headaches.org

National Institutes of Health Neurological Institute and
National Institute of Neurological Disorders and Stroke
P.O. Box 5801, Bethesda, Maryland 20824 / 800-352-9424

Other Organizations

Food and Drug Administration Office of Consumer Affairs
5600 Fishers Lane, Rockville, Maryland 20857-0001
888-INFO-FDA or 888-463-6332

National Brain Injury Association Inc.
105 North Alfred Street, Alexandria, Virginia 22314
703-236-6000 / fax: 703-236-6001

National Health Information Center
P.O. Box 1133, Washington, D.C. 20013-1133
800-336-4797 or 301-565-4167

National Trigeminal Neuralgia Association
P.O. Box 340, Barnegat Light, New Jersey 08006
609-361-1014 / fax: 609-361-0982 / e-mail: tna@csionline.net

O.U.C.H.
(Organization for Understanding Cluster Headaches)
3225 Winding Way, Round Rock, Texas 78664
e-mail: ouch@ouch-us.org

Alternative Therapy Organizations

American Academy of Medical Acupuncture
4929 Wilshire Boulevard, Suite 428, Los Angeles, California 90010
323-937-5514

Association for Applied Psychophysiology and Biofeedback

10200 W. 44th Avenue, Suite 304, Wheat Ridge, Colorado 80033

303-422-8436 / fax: 303-422-8894 / e-mail: AAPB@resourcenter.com

National Institutes of Health

National Center for Complementary and Alternative Medicine

NCCAM Clearinghouse, P.O. Box 7923 Gaithersburg, Maryland 20898

888-644-6226 or 301-519-3153 / fax: 866-464-3616

e-mail: info@nccam.nih.gov

Resources for All Headache Sufferers

Newsletters

HeadWay: The Migraine Newsletter (Free to migraine sufferers)

P.O. Box 29169, Shawnee Mission, Kansas 66201-9169

NHF Headlines (National Headache Foundation bimonthly newsletter)

820 N. Orleans, Suite 217, Chicago, Illinois 60610-3132

888-NHF-5552 or 773-388-6399

Books

Recommended by the National Headache Foundation:

10 Simple Solutions to Migraine, Dawn Marcus. M.D. New Harbinger Publications, Inc., 2006.

100 Questions and Answers about Migraine, Katherine A. Henry and Anthony P. Bossis. Jones and Bartlett Publishers, Sudbury, Massachusetts, 2005.

Check-up Chart Migraine Journal and Workbook, V.R. Quinn. Concise Concepts, LLC., 2004.

Conquering Headache, Alan M. Rapoport, M.D., and Fred D. Scheftell, M.D. Blackwell Science, Inc., 1997.

Coping with Your Headache Problems, Seymour Diamond, M.D. and Mary Franklin Epstein. International Universities Press, 1988.

Headache and Diet: Tyramine-Free Recipes, Seymour Diamond, M.D., Diane Francis, and Amy Diamond Vye. International Universities Press, 1990. (Available from the National Headache Foundation at 800-843-2256.)

Headache Free: A Personalized Program to Stop Migraine, Cluster, Sinus, Tension, Menstrual, and Rebound Headaches, R.K. Cady and K. Farmer. Bantam Books, Inc., 1995.

Headache Help: A Complete Guide to Understanding Headaches and the Medicines That Relieve Them, Lawrence Robbins, M.D., and Susan S. Lang. Houghton Mifflin, 1998. (Available from the National Headache Foundation at 800-843-2256.)

Headache Relief: A Comprehensive, Up-to-Date, Medically Proven Program That Can Control and Ease Headache Pain, Alan M. Rapoport, M.D., and Fred D. Scheftell, M.D. Simon & Schuster, New York, 1991.

The Hormone Headache: New Ways to Prevent, Manage, and Treat Migraines and Other Headaches, Seymour Diamond, M.D., Bill Still, and Cynthia Still. MacMillan, 1995. (Available from the National Headache Foun-dation at 800-843-2256.)

Living Well with Migraine Disease and Headaches: What Your Doctor Doesn't Tell You ... That You Need to Know, Teri Robert. Collins, New York, 2005.

Managing Your Headaches, Mark W. Green, M.D. and Leah M. Green, M.D. Springer-Verlag New York, 2001.

Managing Your Migraine: A Migraine Sufferer's Practical Guide, Susan L. Burke and Fred D. Sheftell. Humana Press, 1994.

Migraine and Other Headaches, William B. Young and Stephen D. Silberstein. Demos Medical Publishing, Inc., 2004.

Migraine: Beating the Odds: The Doctor's Guide to Reducing Your Risk, Richard B. Lipton, M.D., Lawrence C. Newman, M.D., and Helene MacLean. Perseus Books, 1992.

Migraine: The Complete Guide, the American Council for Headache Education, with Lynne Constanine and Suzanne Scott. Delta, 1994.

Migraine: What Works! Joseph Kandel, M.D. and David B. Sudderleth, M.D. Prima Publishing. (To order, call 800-844-7880.)

Migraines: Everything You Need to Know About Their Cause and Cure, Arthur Elkind. Avon, 1997.

Relief from Chronic Headache, Antonia Van Der Meer. Dell, 1990.

Taking Control of Your Headaches: How to Get the Treatment You Need, Paul Drucko, Ph.D., et al. Guilford Press, 1995. (Available from the National Headache Foundation at 800-843-2256.)

TMJ: Its Many Faces, Wesley Shankland, D.D.S., M.S. Anadem Publishing, 1998.

Treating the Headache Patient, R.K. Cady and A.W. Fox. Marcel Dekker, 1995.

Books: Alternative Therapy

Headaches: An Alternative Medicine Definitive Guide, Robert Milne, M.D., Blake More, and Burton Goldberg. Alternativemedicine.com, 1997.

The Homeopathic Treatment of Children, Paul Herscu, M.D., North Atlantic Books, Berkeley, 1991.

The Honest Herbal: A Sensible Guide to the Use of Herbs and Related Remedies, V.E. Tyler. Haworth Press, Binghampton, New York, 1993.

Yoga Therapy for Headache Relief, Peter Van Houten and Rick McCord. Crystal Clarity Publishers, Nevada City, California, 2004.

Guided Imagery Resources

Preparing for Surgery: A Mind-Body Approach to Enhance Healing and Recovery, William Deardoff, Ph.D. and John Reeves, Ph.D. New Harbinger Publications. (To order, call 800-748-6273.)

Cleveland Clinic Section of Health Psychology
9500 Euclid Avenue, Desk P57, Cleveland, Ohio 44195
216-444-5816 or 800-223-2273, ext. 45816
(relaxation tapes and compact discs)

Resources for Children and Adolescents

The Brain Pack: An Interactive, Three-Dimensional Exploration of the Mysteries of the Mind, Ron Van Der Meer and Ad Dudink. Running Press, 1996.

Headache and Your Child, Seymour Diamond, M.D. with Amy Diamond. Fireside Books/Simon & Schuster, New York, 2001.

Headaches, Mary Kittredge. Chelsea House Publications, 1986. (For school-aged children to young adults.)

Headaches in Children, *A Practical Informative Guide for Parents, Teachers and Paramedical Personnel*, Leonardo Garcia-Mendez, M.D. Lemar, 1996. (Available from the National Headache Foundation at 888-643-5552.)

Stress Reduction

Cool Cats, Calm Kids: Relaxation and Stress Management for Young People, Mary L. Williams and Dianne O'Quinn Burke. Impact Christian Books, 1996. (For children age 7 to12.)

Don't be S.A.D.: A Teenage Guide to Handling Stress, Anxiety and Depression, by Susan Newman. Julian Messner, 1991.

Fighting Invisible Tigers: A Stress Management Guide for Teens, Earl Hipp. Free Spirit Publishers, 1995.

Take a Deep Breath: The Kids' Play-Away Stress Book (includes book, clay, and cookie-cutters), Laura S. Shelton, Lawrence E. Shapiro and Bob Beckett. Childswork/Childsplay, 1992.

Tiger Juice: A Book About Stress for Kids, Stewart Bedford. A&S Press, 1981. (For children age 8 to 11.)

What Do Lions Know About Stress? Ali Majid. Life Span, 1996.

You and Stress: A Survival Guide for Adolescence (Self-Help for Kids), Gail C. Roberts and Lorraine Guttormson. Free Spirit, 1991.

Resources for Parents and Teachers

Helping Children Cope with Stress, by Avis Brenner. Health and Co., 1985.

How to Influence Children: A Handbook of Practical Child Guidance Skills, by Charles Schaefer. Jason Aronson Inc., 1994.

How to Talk So Your Kids Will Listen & Listen So Your Kids Will Talk, by Adele Faber. Simon & Schuster, 1995.

Stress and Your Child: Helping Kids Cope with the Strains and Pressures of Life, by Bettie B. Youngs. Fawcett Columbine, 1995.

Your Child: Headaches and Migraine – Practical and Easy-to-Follow Advice, by Maggie Jones. Element Books, 1999.

Other Resources

Relief from Migraine
35-minute video available from the American Council for Headache Education. (800-225-ACHE)

About Robert S. Kunkel, M.D., F.A.C.P.

Dr. Robert S. Kunkel graduated from Mount Union College in Alliance, Ohio, and received his M.D. degree from the University of Pittsburgh. He has been an internist at Cleveland Clinic for more than forty-five years, devoting the last forty years to the treatment of patients suffering with headaches. Dr. Kunkel was instrumental in establishing the Headache Clinic at Cleveland Clinic and currently serves as a consultant in the Headache Section of the Department of Neurology. He has published close to 100 papers and book chapters on headache and related subjects, and is the co-editor of a textbook on headache.

Dr. Kunkel has delivered hundreds of lectures and talks on the subject of headache, and appears frequently as a guest on radio and television programs. He served a term as president of the American Headache Society (formerly the American Association for the Study of Headache) and was the United States representative to the International Headache Society's first Classification Committee from 1985 to 1988. He was president of the National Headache Foundation from 1995 to 2005 and remains active on its board of directors. He also was president of the Ohio Headache Association, a group he helped to found, from 2000 to 2005.

Index

Cleveland Clinic Press

Cleveland Clinic Press publishes nonfiction trade books for the medical, health, nutrition, cookbook, and children's markets. It is the mission of the Press to increase the health literacy of the American public and to dispel myths and misinformation about medicine, health care, and treatment. Our authors include leading authorities from Cleveland Clinic as well as a diverse group of experts drawn from medical and health institutions whose research and treatment breakthroughs have helped countless people.

Each Cleveland Clinic Guide provides the health-care consumer with practical and authoritative information. Every book is reviewed for accuracy and timeliness by Cleveland Clinic experts.

For more information, visit www.clevelandclinicpress.org.

Cleveland Clinic

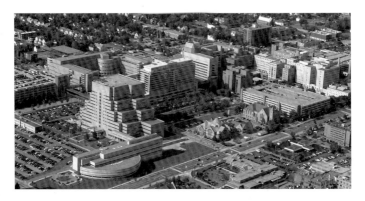

Cleveland Clinic, located in Cleveland, Ohio, is a not-for-profit multispecialty academic medical center that integrates clinical and hospital care with research and education. Cleveland Clinic was founded in 1921 by four renowned physicians with a vision of providing outstanding patient care based upon the principles of cooperation, compassion, and innovation. *U.S. News & World Report* consistently names Cleveland Clinic as one of the nation's best hospitals in its annual "America's Best Hospitals" survey. Approximately 1,500 full-time salaried physicians at Cleveland Clinic and Cleveland Clinic Florida represent more than 120 medical specialties and subspecialties. In 2006, patients came for treatment from every state and 100 countries. For more information, visit www.clevelandclinic.org.